Recovery in Mental Health Nursing

Recovery in Mental Health Nursing

Edited by Nick Wrycraft and Alison Coad

Mc Graw Hill Education

Open University Press

Open University Press
McGraw-Hill Education
8th Floor
338 Euston Road
London
NW1 3BH

email: enquiries@openup.co.uk
world wide web: www.openup.co.uk

and Two Penn Plaza, New York, NY 10121-2289, USA

First published 2017

A catalogue record of this book is available from the British Library

ISBN-13: 978-0-33-526344-8
ISBN-10: 0-33-526344-5
eISBN: 978-0-33-526345-5

Library of Congress Cataloging-in-Publication Data
CIP data applied for

Typeset by Transforma Pvt. Ltd., Chennai, India

Contents

List of figures and tables

List of editors and contributors

Kike Abioye graduated with a first class (Hons) in B.Sc. Nursing (Mental Health) from Anglia Ruskin University and currently practices in an inpatient Acute Assessment Unit (AAU) in Cambridgeshire and Peterborough NHS Foundation Trust.

Melanie Cotter qualified as a registered mental health nurse from Anglia Ruskin University in 2015, with a first class honours degree, and gained the Vice Chancellors award for the best academic performance in pre-registration nursing. Melanie has a specialist interest in females with personality disorder, and currently works in acute inpatient mental health nursing.

Alison Coad is an Occupational Therapist and Cognitive Behavioural Therapist specialising in the treatment of children and young people. She works in London and Suffolk.

Allen Senivassen is a retired Senior Lecturer from Anglia Ruskin University and specialises in clinical leadership and group clinical supervision. He now works as Education Facilitator for Essex Partnership University Trust with a particular focus on coaching and promoting evidence based practice.

Adrian Thackeray obtained a Vice Chancellor's award and first class honours when qualifying as a Registered Mental Health Nurse with Anglia Ruskin University. He currently works in clinical practice and is a recovery champion. He guest lecturers on recovery, and has devised modules for recovery colleges.

Nick Wrycraft is a Mental Health Nurse and Senior Lecturer in Mental Health Nursing with Anglia Ruskin University.

Acknowledgements

Thanks to Nick Wrycraft for inviting me to be a part of this project. Thanks too to Tom: your academic journey is an inspiration.

Alison

There are so many people to thank equally, so please do not see this list as being in any order. I am so grateful to Emily and Hamish for keeping me going when times have been as tough as they have lately. Thanks so much to Karen Harris and Richard Townrow from McGraw-Hill: Open University Press for your unswerving support, belief in me and help during the writing of this book, and to Alison for our many motivational chats over a cup of coffee. Also to the wonderful students and colleagues at Anglia Ruskin University, and the staff in clinical practice who have helped to reaffirm to me that recovery exists.

Nick

Introduction

Nick Wrycraft

Many question the value and contribution of theory to practice. The promotion of unhelpful myths, such as the so-called '*theory-practice gap*', has only damaged and undermined attempts to reinforce values-based practice. Arguably we most need theory, where it is most in conflict and at variance with practice. Recovery is important because it is at the centre of mental health nursing and without its principles guiding practice, we could not possibly hope to learn or develop. By reflecting upon recovery and considering what this tells us about practice we can improve and advance as practitioners and people. This book intends to closely link theory and practice and show the key role of values, principles and recovery. If we can trace the links between our personal values and professional principles in practice, then we may find ways to support service users effectively in their recovery.

The motivation for writing this book stems from one question: what is recovery? Asking this same question of different people will elicit widely differing and contrasting responses. This is in spite of recovery being the preferred philosophy within mental health for many years now. The enigmatic nature of recovery has also led to it being regarded as covering everything. As a result, recovery is poorly understood, and often seems to be quite vague. In this book we will look at different understandings of the term, and encourage readers to develop a personal appreciation of what it means. Various perspectives of recovery will overlap, and some shared characteristics will be apparent. Through reading the book, readers will gain a clearer understanding of what is recovery, what it means for them and, indeed, why they are working in mental health nursing, because recovery is fundamental to the purpose of the profession. Using recovery in our own lives will provide numerous benefits and give us an extra sense of commitment and reward in our work.

From a wider perspective, discussing values, principles and recovery is very timely. The outcome of the *Francis Report* (2013) and *The NHS Constitution* (2012) and waves of other documents that have resulted from the Mid-Staffordshire tragedy has produced significant ramifications. There is now a greater emphasis on embracing values as an inherent part of training students and in helping them to gain knowledge and practice skills. This is a much welcomed turn of events. Arguably mental health nursing was already well situated to participate in this debate. Over a decade ago *The 10 ESC* (2004) and *The Essential Shared Capabilities for Practice* (2007) were direct forerunners of a move to promote values-based practice at the heart of our work. Yet the difficulties in embedding these and resistance within practice reinforce the need for greater commitment and support in promoting values in practice.

The book has three sections. In the first section, Chapter 1 discusses what recovery is, and how we can relate this to our personal values. In Chapter 2 we consider how values relate to professional principles and the nature of recovery in mental health nursing. Section 2 is the longest part of the book and considers recovery from a number of contrasting perspectives. We begin by considering the methods that support students in their learning and professional development, looking at how we communicate, interact, listen to and learn from others. Therefore, in Chapter 3 we discuss communication, in Chapter 4 we look at self-awareness and then in Chapter 5 reflection and clinical supervision. The focus then shifts in Chapter 6 to consider the service user's view, with a particular emphasis on people with borderline personality disorder (BPD). Chapters 7 and 8 then look at the perspectives of other professionals and the multidisciplinary team (MDT), before we consider the involvement of families, carers and significant others. Finally in this section we discuss recovery based ideas and taking practice forward in Chapter 9. This chapter neatly ends Section 2 and provides a useful precursor for Section 3 where we look at recovery-based mental health nursing models. Chapter 10 focuses on Barker's *Tidal Model* (2005) and Repper and Perkins' *Psychosocial Model*, while Chapter 11 then outlines the WRAP and PATH approaches to recovery. Both are influential therapeutic tools that aid recovery and prevent relapse. WRAP was developed by Mary Ellen Copeland and draws on her experience as a service user, while PATH was developed by Ron Coleman who, as a service user and survivor of the mental health system, is a long-established and respected voice of expertise by experience. Finally, in Chapter 12 we provide an overview of the politics of recovery. There is often a sense of apathy concerning politics, as though it is *'other people's business'*. Yet due to the often psychosocial nature of mental illness there are numerous overlaps between politics and health. In this chapter we look at how mental health is inexorably related to politics and the pivotal role of recovery-based values in informing practice. Throughout the book there is an emphasis upon illustrating points that are made with practical explanations and case studies.

This book can be used in several ways. First, the intention is to support students in developing their own growth in understanding recovery. Therefore, it can be read from start to finish as a means of immersing yourself in recovery-based ideas. Through learning about this concept and developing a personal appreciation of what recovery is and what it means for you, you may use the book to chart your personal journey as a reflective practitioner. Second the book is a repository of useful sources on recovery, collected together within one volume. In this sense the book gives the opportunity for practitioners who are interested in recovery to encounter many common ideas as they read through, linked together through the themes of recovery and recovery values and principles, which are discussed. A further use is that the book reflects the state of recovery now. I believe that practice and theory are inextricably linked and that recovery is an innately political notion. These ideas are expounded upon in detail in Chapter 12, yet are replete throughout the whole work. Developing an appreciation of the inherently political nature of mental health nursing will further enhance your sense of values and principles and see further in this important role.

Section 1

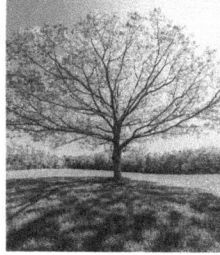

The origins of recovery

1 An understanding of recovery

Nick Wrycraft

Introduction

Recovery represents a whole philosophy and set of beliefs about the world and how it works. If we are to develop an insightful understanding of what recovery means, then it is necessary to apply it to ourselves personally, which can be challenging, and make us question things we previously took for granted. Professional practice can also present challenges, which sometimes appear to undermine our ideals, and it can be tempting to abandon recovery as a desirable but ultimately unworkable dream.

For example, on busy wards that may be relying on bank staff to function, the notion of actively engaging service users in collaboratively planning care may seem to be desirable but loses out in a choice between priorities with the need to carry out observations and just keep everyone safe. It is exactly these dilemmas, and many others like them, which can be seen as the pitfalls of practice highlighting the limitations of recovery.

Yet rather than giving up on recovery, it is still possible to welcome these challenges, and regard them as part of the process of developing a personal understanding that integrates theory and practice. This is where developing personal values can come into play. Reflecting upon our personal values will establish the basis of a deeper understanding of recovery that can be applied in practice, and helps us maintain personal resilience. It also will help us to improve how we support service users. In the early part of this book we explore what recovery is but also what values are and how these make an effective recovery approach possible.

This chapter examines the origins of the concept of recovery in mental health, and considers the meaning of this term before contrasting this view with a traditional or medical approach. Next we look at the personal attributes that are consistent with a recovery-based approach by looking at what values are, and reflecting upon how they feed into our understanding of recovery and mental health.

By the end of this chapter we will have:

- discussed a definition and understanding of the concept of recovery;
- identified key ideas and concepts within the process of recovery;
- considered and reflected upon our personal values.

An understanding of recovery

The concept of recovery began to emerge in the 1980s, with its origins in the treatment of addictions, and the promotion of self-agency and supporting people to take responsibility in moving forward. Patricia Deegan (1988) emphasized the significance of lived experience. Just seeing 'the problem' in isolation fails to understand the full experience, including many of the contributing factors but also many possible sources of support and opportunities for therapeutic progress and growth. Deegan began to think of the experience of mental illness as the same as those in treating addiction. She began to see mental health problems not solely as a 'medical' issue but instead saw it was like other life experiences that can be distressing but at the same time valuable learning experiences in their own right (see the Psychosocial Model of Repper and Perkins in Chapter 10).

The work of Ron Coleman has also been highly influential. His view developed as a result of years as a mental health service user. Coleman identifies a sense of frustration with existing mental health services, highlighting the lack of collaboration with the service user, the punitive as opposed to therapeutic use of legislation to *contain* rather than *care for* the service user, and the limited range of therapeutic options available. In a personal account of his experiences, he identifies the goal of treatment as being to dampen out symptoms (in his case, hearing voices) with medication to the point that his quality of life was severely diminished. He describes being heavily sedated with prescribed medication and permanently tired, and feeling like he was living in slow motion, or in a dream. Coleman (2012) felt that the quality of life afforded by conventional medical treatment and medication was nowhere near adequate. He argued for service users to become more involved in their care, and take much greater responsibility for their recovery.

Rather than the goal of treatment being to remove or subdue voices, Ron Coleman pioneered the Hearing Voices peer support movement in the UK and, alongside Marius Romme and Sandra Escher (2000), who advocated professionals working with service users' hearing voices, opened up other avenues of therapeutic working . Within this broader perception of mental healthcare an increased quality of life for the service user is possible, and we can begin to talk about service users experiencing genuine recovery as opposed to the symptoms simply being subdued. The possibility of working with voices therapeutically, the work of the Hearing Voices network and peer support for service users from other service users has become a much valued mainstay of contemporary mental health care.

Recovery is based on the belief that the experience of mental illness is intensely personal, individual, and different for everyone (Slade, 2009). Therefore two people might experience depression and their symptoms are described in the same way, yet how they understand the experience, and the impact of it upon their lives can be utterly different. As a consequence, the therapeutic approach that is taken will vary, and has to differ depending on the individual. Correspondingly, the service user needs to have input at all stages of their care;

there is a significant emphasis upon the shared nature of care, with the service user an equal participant in the care process. A recovery-based approach emphasizes and actively values the lived experience of the individual.

By far the most frequently cited source defining recovery is Anthony's article, which sees recovery as:

> a deeply personal, unique process of changing one's attitudes, values, feelings, goals, skills, and/or roles. It is a way of living a satisfying, hopeful, and contributing life even with limitations caused by illness. Recovery involves the development of new meaning and purpose in one's life as one grows beyond the catastrophic effects of mental illness.
>
> (Anthony, 1993: 527)

Exercise

Consider which are the most important words and key phrases from the above quote.

Now write down an understanding of the quote in your own words. You do not have to capture everything, just the main points that you feel are important.

Now reflect on your thoughts.

1 Do you agree with Anthony's (1993) view of recovery?
2 If not, then what are your reasons?
3 What else might you add?

Within recovery the experience of mental illness might lead to the person's life taking a different course than they would otherwise have chosen. For many, an important part of their recovery is the process of reconciliation with the losses, but also the gains and crucially the differences that have been experienced as a result of mental illness.

Recovery regards mental health problems as something that cannot be separated from the rest of the person's life. Often after a crisis the person is unsure how to understand the tumultuous and life-changing experience of receiving care. For the person admitted to an inpatient unit in crisis, even if not under a Section of the Mental Health Act (1983 amended 2007), the experience may well be an unexpected and unwelcome episode in their life. It may feel as though that period of time has simply been lost from the timeline of their life, or it may be very difficult to integrate the experience with what has gone before. So it can be reassuring to be able to connect the time spent in crisis with the rest of the person's life, and see continuity, as opposed to the crisis representing an interval, time out, or even time lost. How the service user views their recovery in hindsight and comes to terms with their experience is considered in Chapter 9, where we look at reparation.

Traditional understandings of mental health and illness, which often focus on diagnosis or symptomology, can be unhelpful, because the experience of a mental health problem can only be made sense of in the context of the person's whole life. This makes a great deal of sense, because it is often the case that the apparent cause of a crisis can seem quite innocuous. However, a thorough understanding of the person's wider life experiences will help to identify deep-rooted predisposing factors that have played a contributory role in the person going into crisis. Though often less apparent, these factors are longer lasting, more pervasive and can lead the person to experience ongoing or repeated episodes of crisis. Knowing how to manage, or being aware of these factors can be a useful lever in helping the person avoid relapse(s), and enabling them to take greater control of their mental health in the future. Later in the book in Chapter 11 we discuss the Wellness Recovery Action Plan (WRAP) approach that helps a person to look at their life in these broad terms and to prepare and anticipate the challenges posed by future lapses in their mental health. For many the recurrence of familiar feelings that pre-empt a recurrence of mental illness, and the anticipation of the loss of control that in the past may have followed on from this, increase their anxiety and fear, and in turn make the likelihood of relapse more likely. The more detailed that the relapse prevention plans (and the WRAP approach) are in outlining preventative measures to take in any given situation, the better prepared the person will be to access help and avoid deteriorating further than is absolutely necessary.

Furthermore, within recovery there is an emphasis on collaborative working, sharing power and decision making wherever possible between mental health services and the service user. This can involve accessing and seeking links with other people within the family and social network, and optimizing the service user's choice at all stages of care, whether in complete health or crisis. This aspect of recovery runs counter to the risk-averse culture that pervades mental health services. Often information is withheld or not disclosed without good reason other than concerns that this might represent a conflict of interest. Where in doubt, there is a tendency to withhold information or to err on the side of caution and this can impede open and recovery-focused working.

Recovery also involves the notion that progress will be made at different rates for different individuals, and what works for one person may not for another. In spite of much scientific research, due to the wide range of contributing factors, the causes of mental ill health remain elusive, and in many cases are due to a complex combination of biopsychosocial aspects. Therefore, recovery involves the service user establishing their own meaning and understanding of their experience. Recovery applies not only to how we understand the experience of mental illness but also to the response offered by services. We need to place an emphasis on the person's practical and emotional strengths and resources, and focus on how learning from a crisis equips the person in moving forward with their life, including responding to further episodes. In Chapter 2 we look at the specific principles of a recovery-based approach. Among the various models of recovery, it is worth noting that the most commonly occurring principle is that of developing and maintaining hope, and it is perhaps this attribute that we ought to place at the centre of our practice.

A contrast between recovery and the traditional model

Recovery represents a significant departure from previous approaches to mental health. Not too long ago, service users were encouraged to be unquestioningly compliant with decisions made about them, and not to take an active role in their care or treatment. In spite of major strides in recent years, and the adoption of recovery as the prevailing philosophy informing care, more progress needs to be made to actively and genuinely implement this approach in the care of service users.

What is known as the traditional approach could be categorized as the medical model, but also a general attitude and set of values and beliefs upon which institutional care was organized and run. While this is not to suggest that the medical profession still practises in an unenlightened manner (many doctors, for example, are active and vocal supporters of recovery), the traditional approach has a number of features that do not promote collaborative working in partnership with service users but is instead expert-led and dominated by the opinions of professionals.

Recovery stands as a contrast with traditional views of mental illness, both in how it is understood, and also the approach in practice. For example, recovery perceives mental health problems as something that may be overcome, regardless of the person's clinical progress or continuing symptoms. A sense of mental well-being, quality of life and satisfaction can be achieved in spite of the periodic recurrence of symptoms, or mental health problems on an ongoing and consistent basis. In contrast, a traditional view measures success on the extent to which symptoms of the mental health problem desist, and in terms of clinical outcomes, so continuation of the problem may eventually exhaust treatment options. Within this view many people with ongoing mental health issues may understandably feel rejected by the healthcare system as they can never return to full health. In the past, mental health has been regarded pessimistically as an area of health for which there are few or limited treatment options other than medication that may or may not work. Unsurprisingly, therefore, service users feel a loss of esteem, diminished self-worth, and perhaps even a loss of any hope at all in the face of these circumstances. Yet as we have mentioned, hope is at the heart of recovery and our practice as mental health nurses.

The medical approach is also characterized by seeking to identify mental health issues in terms of symptoms, which are then collected together to contribute to a diagnosis in the *Diagnostic and Statistical Manual of Mental Disorders 5* (DSM) (2013) or the *ICD-10 Classification of Mental and Behavioural Disorders* (1990). Although diagnosis can be very helpful, certainly in terms of identifying suitable medication and appropriate psychological treatment modalities, this is one aspect of care as opposed to the prime focus. Recovery regards these same clinical features as inextricably part of the person but not something that can be separated or seen in isolation and still retain the same meaning. The notion of focusing only on certain specific symptoms or features fails to understand the person in their full complexity and entirety as a biopsychosocial entity. Instead, our mental, physical and sociological health are all intricately connected and mutually influential.

Within a traditional approach, following on from diagnosis comes the prescription of appropriate medication, or other evidence-based treatment, for example, cognitive behavioural therapy (CBT). While in many cases this is undoubtedly valuable in terms of reducing distress and promoting mental well-being, from a recovery-based perspective, medication and psychological treatment are just one part of a comprehensive plan of care, as opposed to the main component. A recovery-based approach, while recognizing the value of these interventions, would see them acting alongside other measures focused on the person's independent coping resources (see Table 1.1).

Finally, although much less in vogue now (perhaps due to the rise of information technology and the availability of vast amounts of health information via the internet), traditionally there has been a dominance of professional expertise, which has had a tendency to limit the extent of involvement of service users in their own treatment. Often this has limited the service user's sense of choice and empowerment within their care, and stifled their progress. Within recovery, a central attribute is the participation of the service user at all stages of their care, and transparency and equality between the practitioner and service user; the service user becomes their own expert, as they have the best knowledge of their situation. This can be challenging, and there may be a temptation on the part of the healthcare professional to compel the person to make the choices that we believe will be 'good for them'. However, it is essential

Table 1.1 Contrast of the traditional and recovery approach

Medical model	Recovery
Sees illness as being curable and measured against objective criteria for recovery, such as improvement or cessation of symptoms	Sees mental illness as something that can either be overcome, be an ongoing problem, or may recur, with no one outcome better than another, just different. Looks at subjective recovery and how the person feels
Collects symptoms or features in order to diagnose in accordance with the ICD or DSM	Sees individual features as just part of the overall presentation that we need to see in order to understand issues
Predominantly relies on medication, though may use other evidence-based treatment such as CBT	Recognizes the value of evidence-based treatments, but within a wider programme of care and within a comprehensive biopsychosocial approach
Sees the healthcare practitioner as expert	Promotes an equal relationship, perhaps with the service user as expert

that the person takes the lead in making not only the choice but also by leading the process by which choice is made. Sometimes, in an effort to stretch resources, healthcare professionals want to move the service user's care forward at a faster pace than the service user is willing or able to manage. It is worth bearing in mind that to avoid rapid relapses or setbacks, it is necessary to make changes that will be sustainable, and these are often not achieved quickly. Instead goals need to be carefully worked towards if we are to keep hold of the gains that have been made.

Exercise

Reflecting on the above, which do you feel is more in accordance with your approach to practice, the medical model or recovery, or vice versa? List the reasons why you might reach this conclusion.

Looking at this list, are there any areas that you might want to change in your practice to work in a more recovery-oriented manner? What would be the advantages of this?

While we have discussed the medical model approach and recovery as almost contradictory, they are not so clearly opposed in practice and may often be seen to be working together. In Chapter 7 we look at working with other disciplines and agencies to consider how working with other approaches to practice can be successful. It is helpful for a medical diagnosis to be made, and for service users to be prescribed the correct medication to alleviate their distress and to stabilize acute symptoms. For many people medication offers an invaluable support. However, at the same time this needs to be offered in addition to a supportive, personalized plan of care in which the service user's needs and priorities are listened to and that reflects the person's long-term goals and aspirations.

Furthermore, the service user needs to be aware of and able to access resources to keep them well, contingency plans need to be in place in the event of relapse, and services need to be available in the long term for service users with ongoing mental health needs. It is noticeable that mental health services are often designed around what are perceived as temporary needs of service users. For example, access and crisis teams are on hand for community-based crisis, while the inpatient sector provides acute beds and for those under Sections of the Mental Health Act (1983, amended 2007). Yet there are very limited resources available to support service users with their needs when not in crisis. The striking rates of relapse for most major mental health problems (Wrycraft, 2015) suggest that there is a lack of recovery-focused thinking and long-term planning that would both reduce the distress for service users and their families and significant others, and at the same time ensure that mental health services worked better to effectively address the needs of service users.

In everyday practice in mental health settings, it is noticeable that recovery is still not really prominent in practice, even among mental health nursing students, who, as Stacey and Stickley (2012) suggest, might be expected to be more idealistic and more receptive to these ideas. The possible reasons include:

- the high profile of evidence-based practice means that the scientific aspects of care and specific interventions are easier to measure, and more likely to appeal to managers and commissioners as opposed to the whole recovery approach;
- reductions in resources and demands for example to see high volumes of service users mean that there is less time for clinicians to spend individually with service users to practise the recovery approach;
- the very clear remits of services, use of standardized assessment tools and means of recording care mean that there is limited scope and flexibility for recovery-oriented practice;
- many service users are cared for under a section of the Mental Health Act (1983, amended 2007) and/or in secure environments, and these custodial settings impose significant boundaries and negative influences on the thera-peutic relationships between staff and service users and stifle creativity in planning care;

Can you think of any others?

Among the measures that might ensure students become effectively engaged with recovery are more actively and meaningfully including service user input throughout the pre-registration curriculum, ranging from the interviewing and selection of students, to the content of the pre-registration teaching. In this way service user perspectives would become more integrated within the culture of mental health professionals. However, service user perspectives might also be usefully involved in the planning of mental health services and priority setting, both nationally and locally, so that the services that are provided more closely resemble those that service users need. While sometimes this is happening, anecdotally mental health services often regard the views of service users and service user groups with scepticism, or to be treated with caution. Service users are often seen as unreliable, or unable to give an informed opinion if asked about their experience.

Q: Do you think service users should be routinely asked about their experience on being discharged, or when their contact with the service ends? What are the reasons for your answer?

A: For: The service user is in a unique position, and has a perspective that professionals, no matter how empathic, cannot fully appreciate. Through asking for service user feedback we might be able to identify consistent themes and suggestions for improving the service to make it more user-friendly.

Against: Often the experience of a mental health problem can be highly emotional, and even if other people might feel that the care was good, due to how they feel, the service user may give detrimental feedback.

Consider the answers above. Are either of them consistent with the principles of recovery?

The reasons for seeking feedback reflect a positive view of service users, which is open and receptive. The reasons against seeking feedback may arise from a paternalistic view of services – one which regards service users with suspicion, and may hint at an oppositional relationship. In terms of the contrast between the traditional approach and recovery, the reasons against seeking feedback belong with the former, in the sense that the professionals regard themselves as the experts. Even for individuals who have received a professional training, no amount of preparation allows one person to see everything. Within a recovery approach, working in a collaborative, inclusive manner that involves the perspective of all of the stakeholders in any situation would seem to be a prerequisite.

From the exercise we have just carried out, it is possible to see that, while often not obvious or routinely acknowledged, we are surrounded by discussions in which there is debate between the traditional and recovery approach. Yet few people would voluntarily identify themselves with a traditionalist approach. In spite of the popular impression we have received, the distinction between these approaches was never as clear-cut as we are sometimes led to believe. For example, the institutionas, classically thought to date from the eighteenth to the mid-twentieth century, is often presented as the epitome of the traditional model. There were undoubtedly numerous abuses of human rights, poor care and neglect. Yet it was also often the case that former service users became attendants, the modern equivalent of which is peer workers; while the work of Joseph Tuke at the York Retreat, which pioneered person-centred care, occurred at the peak of the institutional era (Jones, 1993; Nolan, 1993). Furthermore, the role of the mental health nurse began to develop from the attendants in the institutions. Care in the community has led to a significant evolution in the role, yet the values on which the profession is based and the identity of mental health nursing have endured. Consequently, viewing the traditional medical model and the recovery approach as being diametrically opposed is mistaken. Both are evident in practice and perform particular roles.

In practice, it is worth reflecting on your own attitudes, and those of other practitioners with whom you work, and who may be your mentors, in order to identify the extent to which they reflect recovery-based values and principles. Often these are subtle and difficult to discern and apparent in terms of the attitudes, behaviours, interactions between multidisciplinary teams (MDTs), and choices of interventions made. The example we look at next provides a useful illustration.

Example

A service user who has a history of schizophrenia over many years has been refusing to take their anti-psychotic medication as prescribed. They have been admitted to an inpatient unit on several occasions recently, and sometimes under a Section 2 of the Mental Health Act (1983, amended 2007). In a MDT meeting one community mental health nurse (CMHN) says they have no idea why the service user has stopped taking their medication, and describes the service user as 'non-concordant with treatment', 'undermining their own care plan' and 'not working with the services'. They feel that the solution is to tell the service user that admission is necessary unless they agree to resume taking their medication. Another CMHN asks whether steps have been taken to actually find out why the service user has stopped taking their medication on this occasion, and talk to them see if there are alternatives that might work. The first CMHN responds that this would be great 'in an ideal world' but that currently there is not the time, as the team are confronted with long waiting lists, staff and time shortages, and other competing priorities.

Q: From the brief details supplied above, which approach do you think is most consistent with a recovery-based approach, and why?

- Finding out why the service user has stopped taking medication.
- Strongly suggesting they may need an inpatient admission.

A: All clinical situations are different, and there are no standard responses. What might be right in one situation may not apply in another. It is important that there is an emphasis upon engaging and communicating with the service user in a manner that responds to their individual circumstances, and so the first response seems to be more appropriate. In some cases people are resistant to medical intervention for many reasons including unpleasant side-effects. There are high rates of people admitted to inpatient units due to stopping anti-psychotic medication.

On the other hand, as is the case in the second option, adopting an approach based on organizational issues, such as resource shortages is not appropriate and serves the needs of the service as opposed to those of the service user. To suggest that the service user is undermining their own care plan and not working with the services, when it is not known why they have stopped taking the medication is an assumption, seems to blame the service user, and does not promote engagement and involvement of the service user in their care. The above reflects an outdated attitude, and does not demonstrate a positive perspective of the service user, or commitment to helping them in their recovery.

In this section of the chapter we have looked at the contrast between the traditional model and a recovery-focused approach to practice. This debate is ongoing and is being carried out all of the time in practice. While I have tended to present the two approaches as contrasting, many practitioners are influenced by both approaches and may believe aspects of both. When on practice placements it is worth reflecting on the approaches adopted by your mentors and other staff and how this influences the care of service users.

It is also worth reflecting on our own opinions regarding the traditional and recovery approaches but perhaps more importantly the reasons why we hold these views. Over time, and as a result of gaining in experience sometimes our views change. Often students feel embarrassed when looking at their earlier work because they feel that they have gained so much knowledge over time and in comparison knew so little. But it is well worth remembering who we were and where we began in our emerging understanding of recovery. In this same vein we now continue to look at our values and how these are formed.

Values-based practice

It is often stated that values are important in mental health practice, but with regard to recovery they are essential. Consciously thinking about our values will help us to develop a clearer understanding of what they are, how we embody them in our lives, and how we apply them in practice. This involves looking at our own preconceptions and limitations, which is difficult but necessary. In some cases we may reappraise our values and realize that we hold preconceptions, mistaken assumptions or judgements about others, but the process of realization is valuable in its own right. We consider these issues in more depth in Chapter 4 where we look at recovery and self-awareness and the damage caused by stereotyping and labelling.

To be authentic, values need to be genuine. The closer our professional values resemble those we have personally, the better we will be able to demonstrate these in practice in our work with service users. Our work will seem to fit with our personality. However, it is important that there is some sense of dialogue between our personal and professional values, otherwise we become like robots and lack a sense of personality or an individual approach to our work. As we are learning to be mental health nurses, it is only to be expected that there will be a period of adjustment, perplexity or even feelings of unease or compromise as we encounter issues and dilemmas that are new to us and about which we might not have thought before. In Chapter 2 we develop this notion and discuss principles that we follow, and their relationship to the values which it is felt that mental health professionals ought to embody.

Q: What do you understand the word values to mean?

A: Values are the fundamental beliefs that we hold, and are intimately connected to our hopes, dreams, wishes and aspirations, and the principles according to which we live our lives. Values are evident in how we act and behave towards others and the ideas, actions and activities that we consider to be important and worth prioritizing. Values are the beliefs that we regard as important, and worth defending, promoting and supporting. In many ways they are the point and purpose of life, and at the heart of everything that we do, and give us hope and motivation.

Often people are said to be different in their private life than they are at work. Yet when working with people in a highly interpersonal setting such as mental health nursing and discussing important ethical issues, it is likely there will be some overlap and investment of our personal self within the professional identity. In some cases our personal values might be what has led us to choose to work in mental health nursing.

There is an inherently human element at the heart of practice that involves feeling and emotion. For example, you may encounter a service user who is angry about being compulsorily detained under a Section of the Mental Health Act (1983, amended 2007) and who is at the door of a locked unit asking you to let them out. Alternatively, a person with cognitive impairment says they have to go home to make tea for their children and is distressed and tearful. You are aware that their children are grown up and have their own children. For most readers their response to these scenarios is to feel a sense of care and concern for the emotional distress of the service users, and to want to help, even if this does not involve acquiescing with the service user's wishes. Both of the above situations are typical occurrences in mental health settings yet it is no less traumatic for those that are experiencing them, and ought to be treated as such. Responding in a manner who acknowledges the service user's feelings, and where the mental health nurse recognizes and uses their own emotional response will ensure that service users receive care that is not only appropriate but compassionate.

Genuinely engaging with the service user involves committing yourself, and investing emotional effort and concern. In Chapters 4 and 5 we discuss self-awareness and reflective practice, clinical supervision and learning from experience. This will help you to identify the mechanisms and resources that can sustain your emotional commitment to practice.

Although being motivated from an optimistic perspective and being a caring person are prerequisites for coming into mental health nursing, caring in itself is not enough. Due to the many differing situations that occur in practice, the ability to reflect on practice and adapt our responses to different situations is also essential. Mental health nurses are in a privileged position of responsibility and power. Acting in a manner that demonstrates an awareness of the role, but also takes account of the varying issues and dilemmas of both caring and acting in the best interests of service users, is essential. In different situations the right thing to do will vary. It is not simply about being kind or helpful but also being mindful of an overarching, values-based rationale. Often values help us to both decide and follow through a course of action, and therefore values are a crucial part of mental health practice.

Q: What are your values? Think of one attribute of your personality or characteristic that you prioritize.

A: Often people identify their values as personal qualities, such as:

- honesty;
- integrity;
- loyalty;
- fairness;
- respecting others;
- trusting others and feeling trusted;
- valuing others/feeling valued.

If you hesitated for a minute to consider what your values were, then you are not alone. As discussed above, while values are central to our identity, we rarely take time to consider or reflect upon what these are because they are so inherently a part of us. Values are often talked about as though they are self-evident, but most people struggle to describe what they are. Because we need a little time to even think of what they are, it is easy to assume that our values cannot be changed. Yet if we are not immediately aware of what our values are, then it may also be the case that we are unaware of how our choices impact on others: there is the potential for our values to have unintended effects upon others.

This has particular consequences for mental health nursing, where service users may feel vulnerable and exposed. They are likely to be experiencing low self-esteem, and maybe even a sense of shame, leaving them especially susceptible to feeling judged or being perceived negatively. It is essential that as mental health nurses we have the courage to understand who we really are – to have considered what is important to us, and what attributes we prioritize and feel to be important.

Values are not necessarily set for life, and although those that are established when we are young may be powerful, change is still possible. The situations and people that we encounter as we go through life often serve to test out our values, both personally and also in terms of how we view the world. Therefore, values flow two ways: first, inwardly and in terms of the attributes that we prioritize as an individual, which influences how we act towards others; second, outwardly in terms of our relationship with the external world and those we encounter in life. These are reciprocal exchanges, in that we display positive values in our interactions with others in the hope that they will act in the same way towards us. The philosopher Immanuel Kant (1724–1804) believed that we are virtuous towards one another only because we hope that others would also act the same way towards us. Consequently, we behave in a morally virtuous way out of self-interest, and not because it is the right thing to do in and of itself. It is undeniably the case that many people enter nursing from a sense of altruism, or a desire to do good for others, which in turn engenders a sense of well-being and fulfilment in us. This too may also be seen as self-serving.

Q: Do you think acting towards others in the way you would want to be treated, or caring for others in order to experience a sense of reward is a self-serving motive?

A: Many people do derive a sense of well-being through helping others, which might be seen as selfish in a broad sense. However, if we help others and feel good about it, then everyone benefits, and surely this is a good thing. While the benefit that we gain differs qualitatively from that of the service user, our actions as a caring professional must prioritize what is in the service user's best interests. Satisfaction from a job well done is an important motivation, but the needs of the service user must always come first.

Most people who work in mental health nursing are driven by a desire to work in an area in which they can help others although the rewards are often not obvious or immediate, and we do not receive thanks or gratitude. Therefore, it helps to be very clear in our understanding not only of our values but also why we choose to be in this line of work to begin with. There are many different reasons, and below are some examples:

- Helping from a sense of conviction that it is simply the right thing to do.
- Having worked with people with mental health issues as a support worker, or another area of mental health, and wanting to work in a more responsible role.
- Having a family member, relative or friend who has lived with a mental health problem and has been helped by the mental health services, and wanting to 'give something back', emulate or be like those people who helped at a really difficult time.
- Alternatively having a family member, relative or friend who did not get the help they needed from the services, and so wanting to 'put things right in the future' and make a positive difference.

Many people will have reasons similar to those above for coming into mental health nursing, or others. For many of us there is likely to be more than one reason. It is not necessary to put these in order, but at various times different reasons will be more or less prominent for us. It is important to know why we are working in mental health so that the rewards of the job are consistent with our expectations. This is important to avoid disappointment, or, for example, effort–reward imbalance. Effort–reward imbalance occurs where the practitioner is working hard but perceives there to be an insufficient reward in proportion to their input, whether this is in terms of praise, thanks, promotion or job satisfaction. As there is such a reliance on interpersonal communication as part of the role in mental health nursing, being aware of whether our expectations of rewards through work are being met is important. Otherwise we may not be as motivated as we might be in working with service users and not provide them with the therapeutic support that they deserve.

Exercise

Think about your reasons for wanting to work in mental health, and try and put these into a phrase that effectively describes them and then write it down.

Now re-read your reasons. How might this be a positive motivation?

Are there any aspects that might not be positive? In some cases there might be reasons that may be negative or positive, as our feelings can be hard to predict.

Among examples of reasons that might be positive include 'my grandfather experienced dementia and in the final stages of his illness was cared for by some really compassionate mental health nurses on an inpatient unit. I was always impressed by how caring they were, and though he often got agitated, even when he was very verbally animated they responded to him in such a calming and attentive manner that he felt listened to and reassured. I would like to be like them.' But there may also be mixed feelings related to this positive motivation, for example, 'My concerns might be that working with people with dementia might cause uncomfortable feelings in me about losing my grandfather. Or I may struggle to emulate those nurses, and then not feel confident.'

Also, think about whether there are any questions that require clarification. For example, if you feel drawn to working with people experiencing mental health problems but have no practice experience, seeking employment in mental healthcare, either in the National Health Service or the private sector, as an employee, volunteer or intern will help.

As mental health nursing students it is important to think about how we feel about what we are doing, because this will inevitably influence how we do things. No matter how positive or motivated we feel, there are days when we are not at our best; there may be aspects of the role we do not like doing, or occasions when we wonder if we have the confidence to do it or the skills. This is no bad thing, but instead proves we are human, and it is normal to have doubts or concerns. It is important to listen to these doubts and concerns, be open about them, and discuss and share them with other students, mentors, lecturers and tutors. It is also important to be willing to listen to feedback from other students – their experiences may well provide you with new insights. Having a clear understanding of why we want to be a mental health nurse to begin with provides solid support and reassurance when in doubt, and helps us to persevere through the difficulties. It also helps us to recognize a sense of success or reward.

Exercise

Now think about the reasons for wanting to be a mental health nurse. Write them down. If there is more than one, they do not necessarily need to be in order of priority. Now read the reasons. If another person gave you these same reasons as their desire to be a mental health nurse, what would your thoughts be? What advice would you give them?

One thing to remember is we are all in a state of recovery from life. The motivation to become a mental health nurse is a force that can be positive, but may also have negative aspects that need to be recognized and managed. For example, if I am inspired by having seen care delivered poorly in the past, and I have high beliefs in my own capabilities, I may struggle to work as a part of a team, or to respond constructively when things do not go well. It is important to periodically re-examine our reasons for wanting to become a mental health nurse, and to review where we are in relation to these. In some cases the original reasons will exert less of an influence, or alternatively new reasons may have appeared that reinforce our choices.

Conclusion

In this chapter we have discussed an understanding of recovery and the central tenets of this approach. We have contrasted the medical model and the recovery approach and highlighted elements of both. While recovery is the prevailing model in practice, there is no clear division and often elements of both approaches are used. We then moved on to look at values, and reflected upon how these interlink with principles and our identity as professionals. But also what these might be for us as individuals and how these lead us into mental health nursing. It is important to continue to be aware of how these changes occur for us over the duration of the course.

2 The principles of recovery

Nick Wrycraft

Introduction

This chapter builds upon the understanding of values established in Chapter 1, and looks at principles of recovery in practice. Often values and principles are thought of as one and the same. Values refer to the beliefs that we hold at an individual level and the subjective rules and precepts by which we live our lives, while principles are broader statements of beliefs held by groups or organizations. Often our values predispose us to pursue particular careers: for example, a person with a caring disposition may gravitate towards working in the health professions. Yet as discussed in Chapter 1, we all have different perspectives and motivations that feed into our values. When training as a mental health nurse, therefore, it is necessary to examine and reflect on our values, and consider how these connect with the prevailing principles of the profession. This is an important part of developing your identity as a healthcare professional and person.

We begin the chapter by looking at how legislation dictates the nature of our interactions with service users in practice, and the implications for our values and a recovery approach. Then we consider the principles of recovery more broadly. Throughout this discussion you are encouraged to reflect upon the dilemmas these issues present in your own practice experience. This will enable you to develop your understanding of yourself, but also about mental health nursing and the concept of recovery.

By the end of this chapter we will have:

- considered how principles in practice are guided by legislation and expectations of us as professionals;
- discussed how principles inform a recovery-focused approach;
- reflected on our personal values in relation to the broader principles of recovery in practice.

Legislative principles of recovery

Alongside the Nursing and Midwifery (NMC) Code (2015) in mental health nursing practice, perhaps the most dominant factor guiding practice in mental health nursing is legislation. This imposes an array of obligations and non-negotiable expectations upon our conduct. In this section of the chapter we look at some of the dilemmas we may encounter.

The overriding principle concerning mental health legislation is that any sanction used ought to be the least punitive option for the service user. This is a result of many years of debate, consultation and development of mental health law incorporating the views of professionals, stakeholders and more recently service users. Many specific pieces of legislation are used in practice. Working in accordance with the law also allows little scope for flexibility. Commonly, we work in one of three ways:

– interpreting the law;
– applying the law;
– working in accordance with the spirit of the law.

Approved qualified mental health professionals (AMHPs) alongside other designated professionals are often involved in interpreting whether the Mental Health Act (1983, amended 2007) can be applied. This involves:

– carrying out a suitable assessment;
– consulting as appropriate with the service user, their family and significant others;
– liaising with other healthcare professionals as required by the law, and in conformity with good practice and team-working.

Once a Section of the Mental Health Act (1983, amended 2007) (HM Government, 2007) is imposed, the nursing staff are required legally and ethically to abide by the specific criteria of the relevant Section and we go from applying general principles to conforming to the exact 'letter of the law'. Nursing staff may be tasked with ensuring that the service user does not leave the inpatient unit, and managing the person's leave in terms of where they can go, for how long and who with. Often the service user unsurprisingly resents the limitations imposed on their freedom. This inevitably produces tensions in the relationship between the service user and mental health nurses. Working in these circumstances is challenging, but is perhaps one of the most fulfilling and rewarding parts of the role of being a mental health nurse. This is because of the potential of helping the service user to make a difference at a difficult time in their life.

To understand how a person who does not want to engage feels, but is compulsorily detained, requires empathy and sensitivity. For example, imagine that you are a service user on an inpatient unit and are told that you cannot leave. You may not previously have even wanted to leave, but suddenly this may feel like the thing you most want to do. The unit may then feel like a prison, and somewhere towards which you channel all of your negative feelings. Understanding this viewpoint will help the mental health nurse work with the defensiveness and resistance to treatment that the service user may express.

Being positive and respectful towards the service user is essential, while negotiating over the aspects of their daily life in which the person can gain more freedom is an important therapeutic intervention.

Recovery plays an important part in promoting and empowering the service user even when the person is acutely unwell. Sensitively providing the necessary support to compensate for the deficit, and offering therapeutic support until such time as the person is able to resume control and self-agency, comprise an essential role of the mental health nurse and aspect of recovery. It is important to remember the role of the nurse as to 'do with' as opposed to 'doing for' the service user. Mary Ellen Copeland's Wellness Recovery Action Plan (WRAP) (which is discussed in Chapter 11) takes us further, as her work serves to alleviate some of the trauma of the complete loss of independence and confusion that can beset the person in crisis. The WRAP represents a way of reducing the effects of losing autonomy, making it easier to recover from crisis and ensuring there is a route back to normality and a sense of equilibrium. In response, the mental health nurse needs to be able to discreetly ascertain when to take control for the person, but also at other times to encourage the person to take control for themselves. In some cases therapeutic risk is necessary, and at other times our hands are tied and we have no scope for choice due to the requirements of legislation.

Decisions should not be taken alone, however, and in most cases the mental health nurse works as part of a multidisciplinary team (MDT), which shares responsibility for care of the individual and in which these conversations can be undertaken. It is essential for all team members to be fully aware of the factors that are active within the situation, and to understand the ways in which the roles of different team members interact. In Chapter 7 we discuss the MDT, which is a crucially underestimated aspect of the work of not only mental health nurses but also all professionals working in this area.

Often when on placement on an inpatient unit, students will simply 'join in' with the work. Supporting service users in their daily lives, helping them achieve personal goals as identified in their care plans and attending MDT meetings seem to be a natural activity. There is a general forwards-directed momentum of care that propels most service users back into the community. Even where there are setbacks, there is a reformulation and emphasis on improvising an alternative set of goals for the service user's care. However, recovery does not happen by accident. It is worth reflecting on the often complex nature of the relationship that the service user has with the mental health services. Sometimes this has an unpromising start but is worth persevering with and being patient. If the person is compulsorily detained, there will inevitably be feelings of resentment and hostility, as they have not agreed voluntarily to the admission. For some, the mental health services may represent an unwelcome reminder of their mental health problem, but the service user needs to receive positive opportunities to engage with the mental health services to begin to progress. Being accommodating and available are prerequisites in these situations as shown in Case Study 2.1.

Case Study 2.1   Example 1

A service user in his twenties has a history of schizophrenia and substance use, and repeated compulsory inpatient admissions. He has not been taking his anti-psychotic medication, seems distracted and is not engaging with anyone or anything, but is responding animatedly to apparently invisible stimuli, and as a result has been admitted to the inpatient ward. He seems to be unaware of his surroundings, does not respond to other people, and has been neglecting his self-care. Although not resisting care, he requires prompting, and in some cases support to carry out most basic tasks and activities of daily living. A mental health nurse will:

- talk to the person, communicating and asking questions, even if the person does not reply;
- involve them in their care and work as collaboratively as possible;
- explain procedures and seek consent for every interaction;
- work at a measured pace, rather than rushing;
- develop a better understanding of the person beyond these sketchy details so we know the person and not a stereotypical collection of details.

What other considerations can you think of that might support the person?

Exercise

Looking at Case Study 2.1, have there been instances in your practice placements where you have seen all of these elements apparent in the care that was given?

How did you feel to be participating in care of this kind?

Write a brief reflective account of one particular situation where you took part in care that was especially service user-focused and you felt it was particularly good.

Alternatively, have you been on placements where you have felt that these elements were not present? Again, write a brief reflective account of one instance where the care was lacking, identify how and in what ways, and consider how more recovery-focused care might be promoted.

It is an important role of the mental health nurse that through our actions and engagement we demonstrate respect for the person, actively collaborate and seek to involve them in partnership with their care, see meaning in their life and value them as an individual. This reflects a shared sense of purpose consistent with recovery, and in terms of permitting the person to do what they can but offering support where necessary. Often the goal of healthcare practitioners in promoting independence is assumed to mean complete autonomy. The service user does not have to be at a certain level of functioning and mental well-being in order to experience recovery. A recovery approach will help to guide the actions taken by nursing staff. The aim is to identify a positive and personal focus that optimizes the person's capabilities and potential consistent with their goals and aspirations, even where progress might not be evident in objective or clinical measures. Instead, care is evaluated using a more flexible but still evidence-based criteria.

Care that does not use the recovery approach might be seen as task-based. In this sense we simply provide support to compensate for the person's perceived level of deficit, without an emphasis on promoting independence and empowerment. Often because a person cannot carry out one activity, it is tempting to assume that they cannot perform others that require an equivalent level of skill or competency. This does not demonstrate a person-centred focus, is complacent and can lead to the service user losing independence and becoming de-skilled. In some cases a person may be able to complete a task on some days but not on others. For example, a person with dementia may be able to eat independently sometimes but not at other times. The person's ability may fluctuate, or they may struggle when tired or fatigued. Sometimes people who are depressed may experience differing levels of motivation through the day and their ability to function may be intermittent. Communicating with the person about their wishes regarding their care represents social contact and inclusion of the most fundamental kind. Often people in care are prone to depression, low mood and loss of esteem.

Q: Is it possible that a person with advanced dementia can still experience recovery?

A: An important feature of recovery is that it is not dependent on the person making improvements that are objectively measurable in clinical terms. Recovery pertains to subjective quality of life, the person's needs being met, and their feelings valued and being able to engage in meaningful social interaction. Often these are important functions of mental health nurses who work with people with dementia. As we discuss in Chapter 3, communication is not just the purpose of imparting and receiving information. Instead, there is also a social value in terms of recognizing others, sharing impressions, fears and concerns, but also in offering reassurance, support and most importantly care. Recovery therefore should not only fundamentally inform our approach, but should also be an essential part of the mental health nurse's actions, regardless of the nature or severity of the problem, or the likely prognosis.

Q: Think about the two examples we have just discussed; one of a person with schizophrenia and substance use issues, and the other a person with dementia. Did thinking of one person with schizophrenia, and then needing to rapidly switch and think of another person with dementia require you to take a moment to think about your perceptions? Why might this be the case?

A: We are often prone to forming stereotypes and preconceptions that conform to labels and values. In Chapter 4 we discuss stereotypes in more depth, and examine this concept. However, in the above examples a point worth considering is that we have widely different expectations from these mental health issues. Even mental health professionals are prone to labelling and stereotyping. We can never remove our tendency towards forming preconceptions but it is important to be aware of how they may influence our practice.

Exercise

Try monitoring your own thinking, and look for instances where you are stereotyping. This may be in daily life, or on placement. Once you identify a stereotype, consider why, and on what grounds you might make this assumption.

Next, challenge the stereotype. Does the person fit with the set of expectations you have for them?

If not, why not?

What does this add to your learning in moving forward?

How might you approach the same or a similar situation again?

What might be the benefits for you, and those who you come into contact with?

So far we have looked at people with a high level of need that calls for inpatient care. In other circumstances, such as the community, we are still working within the spirit of the law. We are required to seek the service user's agreement to participate in care plans and to engage in treatment. We must take care to explain procedures, possible therapeutic options and the intended effects and possible side-effects of treatment. Working consistently in accordance with the spirit of the law is an essential principle, and we should at all times use the least punitive sanction and avoid taking away personal liberties and freedom. For example, service users with a severe and enduring mental health problem living in the community often relapse and cease taking their medication. Subjectively, the person does not believe their mental health has deteriorated, and then understandably questions why they were taking the medication to begin with. This can mean that the service user is quite solidly convinced that they do not require medication, and that there is no need for them to take it. No matter how effective the therapeutic rapport is with the service user, the mental health nurse has a challenge persuading the person to resume taking medication.

Case Study 2.2   Example 2

Q: Imagine you are a mental health nurse working with a service user in the community who has stopped taking their medication. We know that under specific circumstances in accordance with the Mental Health Act (1983, amended 2007) and if under Compulsory Treatment Order (CTO), the person may be compelled to resume taking the medication if all else fails. Why might we feel there to be an ethical challenge to persuading the person to take the medication?

A: The role of the mental health nurse, and other mental health professionals, emphasizes working therapeutically and caring, as opposed to a custodial or controlling role. Yet as the service user may be resistant to taking medication, we may need to take a firm line in trying to persuade them, and it may feel that we are in a position of almost coercing them that if they do not take the medication they could be compelled to do so. This could be seen as contradicting the values of recovery. However, it could also be argued that the longer-term benefit to the service user's mental health justifies any sense of compromise we might feel there to be in the short term. It is essential to persuade the service user that we are acting sensitively, and recourse to compulsory powers is not used casually. Instead the mental health nurse ought always to seek to develop trust with the service user, as opposed to the coercive use of power.

In this sense our values are influential in how we interpret the principles of recovery. We will all have a unique understanding of recovery, and it will feel and mean something different for each of us. That said, the concept of recovery is underpinned by some common values, beliefs and principles with which most of us would agree. Yet it helps to have an appreciation of our individual perspective on recovery and how we learn about it through our experiences. In making sense of how this adds to what we already know, we need to be able to regularly stop and assimilate new learning, and consider how this is consistent with or challenges our understanding.

Exercise

Think of a situation in which you felt uncomfortable, for example, where care had to be given against the service user's wishes in accordance with the law. This may have left you with conflicting feelings of reluctantly being involved in delivering care that was unwelcome but at the same time knowing that for the longer term good it was necessary. Alternatively, choose something that has preoccupied you or caused you to think and experience some perplexity.

Work through the questions listed and then reflect back on what you have learned about the example, but also what you have learned about yourself.

- What is new, and I did not know before?
- What do I already do that is recovery-focused?
- From practice, what do I find hard to fit with my understanding?
- Is there a conflict between my values and the principles that I practise?
- What do I not agree with?
- What do I need to think more about and reflect upon?

It is necessary to continually reflect on our values and how these stand in relation to the dominant principles in practice. At times this can be emotionally fraught, exacting and difficult. Yet becoming a registered mental health nurse requires that you assume autonomy and personal responsibility for your practice, and so it is necessary for all mental health nurses to consider how their work reconciles with their values. This will involve recognizing and addressing difficulties. Yet reflection often reinforces our sense of purpose as to why we work in mental health at all, and ensures that mental health nurses continue to remain caring and compassionate.

Contrast between values and principles

While there are similarities, values tend to be personal and subjective, and apply to particular ways of acting and behaving within individual relationships. Principles on the other hand are more universal, adhered to by groups, organizations and wider society, and refer to collective beliefs in a variety of situations.

Values say something about us as individuals, and our identity as people. For example, some feel that loyalty is especially important. While this is a positive attribute, and could be seen as being a right and a good thing, other people may prioritize a different value. Often, though, values and principles relate to similar things. For example, values often pertain to moral issues, and are about 'right' and 'wrong'; but characteristics such as honesty are likely to be highly valued by most people, and could therefore be defined as an important principle. Often we work in a particular profession because we share the principles of the organization. For example, I may work in the police force because I believe in justice and the value of enforcing the law. Or I may work in mental health nursing because I want to support people in their recovery. Yet often our professional roles will present us with challenges and situations that rock us back on our heels, and make us reflect upon how our personal values might seem to be challenged by the principles of the organization.

Recovery is not something *done to* the person, but worked towards, and so the role of the mental health nurse is to collaborate jointly with the service user supporting their pathway (Slade, 2009). This is not predictable and will not be the same for any two people. Often the role of the mental health nurse is a coach as opposed to being an expert. Within recovery there is a different perception of the power relations than the traditional approach, with the therapeutic relationship between the service user and mental health nurse being at least equal, or if anything the service user assuming a more prominent role in making decisions about their care wherever possible. On the one hand, the mental health nurse has a more flexible, service user-focused perspective, but this also requires courage, as it means eschewing power and control.

Permitting people the licence to make their own decisions requires confidence, belief in their ability to make their own choices, and a good understanding of boundaries and the grounds on which decisions are made. From the earliest stages it is helpful if therapeutic relationships emphasize the service user's active participation, engagement and decision making. In this respect the mental health nurse works alongside the person, as opposed to acting as an expert. Often therapeutic relationships are not developed explicitly but through subtle and discreet understandings and communications that develop spontaneously. Therefore, communication and cues and simply how we are, can be extremely important. Often our values and beliefs are evident through our outward disposition and demeanour, and in numerous respects with regard to how we behave and communicate with others right down to the choice of individual words.

Especially when we are students, it is easy to become insecure and preoccupied with concern over how we ought to appear. In some cases we can try too hard to cultivate an image. This can seem artificial and lead the service user to feel suspicious of the mental health nurse. Alternatively, simply being blasé and not paying any attention at all to how we are engaging will appear careless and lacking in attentiveness. Instead, adopting an approach where there is awareness of how communication is being carried out, yet still with sufficient spontaneity for this to be natural is more likely to foster a good therapeutic rapport. We discuss this further in Chapter 3.

It is important to consciously focus on making communication comfortable for the service user, even if this involves changing an established pattern. For example, if meetings are always at the team's office, it might not occur to the service user to ask for them to be moved to another more comfortable and convenient location. Being open to suggestions from the service user also helps: there is great potential for learning from the service user and their experience. The therapeutic relationship then becomes a mutual learning experience. This represents a quite significant contrast to traditional approaches that involve the imparting of professional expertise to service users in a didactic manner. Therefore, within the recovery approach, the therapeutic relationship and the basis upon which it is founded require greater consideration than in the traditional approach.

Recovery involves adopting a fundamentally different perspective of practice that requires a significant adjustment to the relationship of power and professional control. This is a courageous but also potentially risky step. It offers the possibility of engaging more meaningfully with service users, yet also presents the challenge of revealing more of ourselves in therapeutic engagement – and being more human, more open and willing to learn alongside the service user. To prepare for the demands of this role it is necessary to be clear on the principles that recovery involves. Understanding and fully adapting to the difference in approach between recovery and the traditional approach may take time, and it is worth exploring this in some detail.

Guiding principles of recovery

In identifying the central principles of recovery, Shepherd et al. (2008) cite Andresen et al. (2003) who identify the key components of a recovery framework. These are:

Hope: This is the most common component of all understandings of recovery, and central to making progress and the basis for all future plans. Within all understandings of recovery, hope is a central feature. It is not enough for service users to have hope on their own but it must be reciprocated by the mental health nurse in their believing in the service user.

- Do you feel hope for your service user and positive about their prospects?
- Where does this belief stem from and what supports this view?
- Does your service user feel hopeful about the therapeutic relationship? *Or are they just going through the motions?*

Often in practice settings people can fall between the gaps. Lack of continuity of care, with different members of staff not carrying out care consistently, or tasks not being completed at the right time or not at all, can lead to the service user gaining the impression that their care is not valued by mental health nurses, even if it is. It is always necessary to ensure we deliver what we promise and that care is consistent. The recovery approach ought to nurture a sense of hope, optimism and reliability and to encourage the service user to identify and strive towards their aspirations.

Self-identity: Building a positive self-image for the service user is a central feature of recovery. Self-image often shifts, and can change and fluctuate, so that while the intention is for it to become better, it may also at times deteriorate. Therefore within the therapeutic relationship it can be helpful to promote a sense of self for the service user, helping the person to build self-regard and a realistic awareness of personal worth together with a resilient and robust sense of personhood. There are many ways in which this can be achieved, and every person will have unique needs. We all meet with disappointments or challenges, and we can learn to recognize our sensitivities, but at the same time it can be hard to change. Consequently, the mental health nurse needs to be patient, have perseverance and belief in the service user and offer consistent support.

Meaning: Refers to gaining a balanced sense of value and quality of life. Living a better life is not about experiencing good luck, things going our way, or undergoing a change of fortune – though these all might help. Many service users experience material and emotional deprivation, and may feel that things can only improve if external factors lead to a change. However, there are many other ways in which life can improve; for example, developing a way of looking at life that allows us to understand the actions of others without feeling a sense of being wounded or hurt; or learning to value ourselves, others and the world around us. We may even begin to understand what we can and cannot influence and take responsibility that may make us view disappointments differently and make everything a bit more bearable. Things do not always need to change a great deal in order to bring about a transformation in how we enjoy and value life. Finding meaning in life may be highly elusive, as it cannot be quantified – it is a unique interpretation for each of us. The mental health nurse also needs to consider their own sense of meaning in life in order to be able to recognize how important this is for the service user.

Personal responsibility: Through self-determination and the person having a sense of agency and control over their life. What we take responsibility for varies widely, and can mean numerous things, for example:

- a job;
- a volunteer;
- a parent;
- pet owner;
- tenancy holder.

Responsibility is often seen as a significant burden. However, taking responsibility is an essential part of assuming a role within society, and the sense of identity and self-worth this entails. Taking responsibility can provide reassurance, and help us gain in confidence, reinforcing our esteem and sense of who we are. We want to be seen by others as a person of worth, not in the shallow sense of image, but in deserving respect and regard. Often becoming a mental health nurse leads us to re-evaluate our sense of responsibility. The role of the nurse brings obligation, accountability and expectations from others. This is a significant expectation and role to live up to, and it can be a challenge to adapt.

The National Standards for Mental Health Practice (2010) identify a range of principles of recovery. These are outlined in Table 2.1.

Table 2.1 Principles informing recovery

Principle	Aspects
Each individual is unique	• Recovery is not about cure but gaining choices for the person to help them lead a meaningful, satisfying life, and for them to feel valued in the community • Recovery is different for everyone and involves social inclusion and quality of life • Places the service user at the centre of their care
Real choices	• Empowers the individual to make choices about their life, and that these need to be meaningful and creatively explored • Supports a strengths-focused approach, and the person taking as much responsibility as they are able to handle • Ensures that there is a balance between the duty of care and providing support, and allowing the individual to take positive risk and access new opportunities
Attitudes and rights	• Listening to, learning from and acting upon the service user's and their carer's views • Promoting and protecting the individual's human and legal rights • Helps individuals maintain and engage in social, recreational, occupational and vocational activities • Promotes hope in the person's future and finding meaning in life
Dignity and respect	• Being courteous, respectful and honest in all communication • Sensitivity and respect for the values, beliefs and culture of each individual • Challenging discrimination and stigma
Partnership and communication	• Recognizing that the person is an expert on their own life and it is necessary to work in partnership with the service user • Prioritizing the sharing of relevant information and communicating clearly • Working in a positive and realistic manner towards achieving the service user's hopes, goals and aspirations

Table 2.1 (continued)

Principle	Aspects
Evaluating recovery	• Recovery is continuously evaluated • The service user can track their own progress • Services demonstrate that they use the service user's experience to inform service developments • Mental health services report on key outcomes that indicate recovery including housing, employment, education and social and family relationship and health and well-being measures

Source: Adapted from National Standards for Mental Health Services (2010).

Exercise

The above can be grouped under three categories, of:

- how our beliefs inform practice
- how we proceed
- what our goals are

Group each of the six principles in Table 2.1 under these three categories:

1. Each individual is unique
2. Real choices
3. Attitudes and rights
4. Dignity and respect
5. Partnership and communication
6. Evaluating recovery

Suggested answers:

- Category 1: How our beliefs inform practice
  1, 4, 5

- Category 2: How we proceed
  2, 4, 5, 6

- Category 3: What our goals are
  3, 5

Q: What led you to make these choices? What do you notice?

Suggested answer: Our beliefs often inform our practice. What we do and our goals flow from our initial beliefs and principles. This produces consistency and a sense of continuity between our actions and our beliefs.

In some cases service users might not want to take an active role in collaborating on their recovery, or they might try to abdicate responsibility to you as the healthcare professional.

Q: Why might some service users not want to take an equal role in the therapeutic relationship?

Possible answers:

- The service user may not be used to a recovery approach, and previous contact with the mental health services may have involved a more traditional or medical model approach.
- The service user may not feel motivated, confident or be used to being given choices and control over their care.
- The service user may feel concerned about making a choice and 'getting it wrong' through a lack of esteem and self-agency or having 'got it wrong' before.

In each of the above situations how might we respond to work in a collaborative manner with service users in each of the scenarios?

- Talking through the therapeutic relationship with the service user and negotiating and defining mutual roles and responsibilities.
- Discussing the service user's lack of motivation openly, and recognizing the possible explanations and reasons, such as where a lack of confidence may stem from – for example, has the service user previously experienced difficulties with the notion of choice or having control? What strategies have been tried in the past, and what worked/didn't work?
- Exploring the notion that there is no such thing as 'making a mistake'. We may make choices or decisions which do not yield the benefits we expect, but every choice offers a learning opportunity, and there may be gains in other areas. Also 'all or nothing' thinking can lead to setting expectations at high/unreasonable levels, which do not reflect the way others may view the situation, or a fair appraisal of the facts.

In Chapter 1 (p. 5) Anthony's (1993) definition of recovery was quoted. This still has relevance and currency today. The article from which this definition comes also identifies a number of principles informing recovery. These include:

Recovery is possible without professional intervention: Often people make improvements in their mental health regardless of the input of mental health services. There are numerous resources independent of statutory mental health services, for example, self-help groups, family, friends and social networks, sports clubs, adult education and churches. These all offer valuable sources of support and can promote mental well-being but without being under the mental health service banner.

Recovery is possible for everyone: Even where mental illness is recurrent or ongoing recovery is possible. Within this concept we are all at a point of recovery. As with the Tidal Model (see Chapter 10), while today our mental health may be at an equilibrium, there is no guarantee that tomorrow the situation will be the same. This means that we live in an inherently unstable world, which may be an unsettling thought. Yet at the same time, when people feel stuck, and believe that life can never be improved, there is the comforting thought that things might change for the better.

Recovery is not linear: Progress is not always in a uniform forward direction. There may be sudden changes, unexpected progress, or alternatively setbacks, or inertia. Recovery does not take equilibrium for granted.

The consequences can be worse than the illness: being deemed to be mentally ill, with the associated loss of rights, opportunity, discrimination and damage to esteem, confidence and self-regard may be a worse blow than the illness itself.

Progress is often achieved by taking responsibility: Becoming aware of and feeling empowered in making changes in one's life and taking responsibility are essential in recovery. This is independent of tackling the conventionally perceived disease process. For many, recovery is as much characterized not just by symptoms improving from a medical perspective but also by regaining control over their life again, and making decisions and choices. Responsibility will differ for us all. For some this might be going back to work, but for others it might mean going back home to live independently or the resumption of taking care of their pets.

Recovery requires that people with mental health problems feel accepted: Feeling a sense of identity, worth and acceptance within family, close relationships and social networks is an important protective factor for mental health and well-being. There also needs to be scope for meaningful employment, occupation, and a sense of making a valued contribution to society. Too often, people with mental health issues are consigned to a life on benefits that can mean a lack of connection to others or society and a feeling of dependence as opposed to acceptance. This situation is often perpetuated by the very services that are meant to help the person, for example, mental health nurses encouraging the service user to lead a very safe but ultimately unadventurous and boring life in order to maintain the equilibrium of their mental health. While the person is not exposed to risk, neither is there any stimulation, challenge, reward or opportunity to build confidence and esteem. Instead it is helpful to promote positive therapeutic risk-taking as a means of realizing possibilities and achieving individual goals and aspirations.

Recovery is continuous: Recovery happens every day, can fluctuate, and is something that can improve or deteriorate. In this sense it is like the experience of life, which for the most part hopefully goes well, yet occasionally and sometimes unexpectedly produces reversals or unfortunate events. These should not

Table 2.2 Themes of recovery

Personal	Contextual
Gaining in confidence and self-awareness and understanding the illness, and participating in relationships and roles that promote social growth	Basic and material needs, for example, accommodation, finances, human rights
Taking responsibility in recovery	The impact of stigma and societal attitudes leading to isolation
Self-management in terms of knowing triggers that precede relapse and coping strategies	Positive, supportive, nurturing and confidence-building relationships
Having a purpose and feeling valued and recognized by others	Support from mental health professionals and mutual and informal networks with peers
For some people gaining in spirituality and cultural wisdom	Treatments such as medication, talking interventions or hospitalization as appropriate that are delivered collaboratively and as part of an informed choice

Source: Adapted from Rethink AstraZeneca (2010).

be shied away from but, although they are difficult and challenging, do help us to learn and develop. Anthony (1993) regards recovery as similar to the process of overcoming these life events in the sense that often how we reconcile ourselves to these changes is different, individual and can be hard to define, yet is nevertheless something that we all endure.

In a research project into what helped or hindered the experience of people with mental health issues in their recovery, seven service user researchers carried out semi-structured interviews with 48 people with lived experience of mental health problems (Rethink AstraZeneca, 2010) (see Table 2.2). The project was funded by AstraZeneca, a drug company; Rethink retained control of all aspects of the research to ensure impartiality of the findings. A total of ten themes were identified, with five each being personal and contextual.

Acceptance, control and *interdependence* were identified as being additional themes running through the contextual and personal issues. *Acceptance* involves coming to terms with oneself with regard to the experience of mental illness, but also changes in lifestyle, expectations and attitudes through a growth in self-awareness. Acceptance was also identified as being connected to gaining self-confidence and well-being, and acquiring a sense of purpose. Participating in mindfulness was also mentioned in terms of acceptance through focus on present experience, which can help to lessen preoccupation with concerns and anxiety.

Loss of *control* was also identified as a significant theme when service users experienced severe and acute mental health issues. Regaining control occurred through self-management and avoiding unhealthy behaviours, such as choosing not to engage with voices.

With regard to *interdependence* the research participants talked about difficulties in relationships, where when unwell there was a sense of dependence on the services, friends and family; yet when being well an enforced assumption of independence could lead to isolation. A means of addressing this dilemma was through gaining a sense of purpose and inclusion by helping others in peer and support relationships (Rethink AstraZeneca, 2010).

The same research also identified some recommendations for mental health practitioners. These include:

–   When someone first becomes unwell, clearly explain what is happening and offer reassurance to the person and their family
–   Put yourself in the person's shoes and empathise
–   Talk to people and hear what they have to say; being honest is likely to engender trust in the therapeutic relationship
–   Respect the person's view, and do not assume that as they are unwell, they do not know what they are talking about
–   Prioritise the person not the paperwork
–   Look beyond the diagnosis, as this does not define the person
–   Adopt a holistic approach that involves all options from medication to talking therapies to other options such as peer support
–   Find ways to empower people and to help them regain control over their lives
–   Encouraging people to help others can help them feel valued and that they have something to offer
–   Seek to involve family and friends as appropriate, and communicate with them and listen to their concerns
–   Be willing to talk about spiritual interests
–   Do not dismiss beliefs, even if they are unusual
–   Being in hospital can be challenging and it is essential to offer hope and treat people with care and respect
–   Give people information about their care and treatment. Find out about other organisations and providers. At the start offer information to questions asked as opposed to giving too much information
–   Peer support can help recovery. Isolation can be reduced by signposting people to local support or self-help groups, or setting one up within the workplace.
(Rethink AstraZeneca, 2010).

Exercise

1   Looking at the above, what aspects particularly strike you?
2   Why might this be the case?
3   What can you take forward that will help you practise in a recovery-focused manner?

Exercise revisited

At the beginning of the chapter we looked at your learning. Looking at the following questions, think about what you have learned.

- What is new, and I did not know before?
- What do I already do that is recovery-focused?
- What do I find hard to assimilate with what I understand to happen in practice?
- What do I not agree with?
- What do I need to think more about and read and reflect upon?

What do you need to do next to advance your learning? Set some goals for:

- What you need to learn.
- How you will achieve this learning.
- When it will be achieved.
- How you will know this learning has been met.
- Further goals for learning.

Conclusion

From Chapter 1, where we looked at personal values, we have expanded the scope of our discussion in this chapter to discuss the principles of recovery. Often in practice we are working within the confines of legislation, and this can be seen as limiting the scope of recovery-based practice. Yet this represents a really good opportunity to develop therapeutic relationships that promote recovery and empowerment of the service user. The relationship between the expectations of professional and legal requirements and our own values is extremely important. We will respond better to unique situations for which there is no guidance and precedent if we know ourselves and how we really feel about the issues with which we are dealing. We then moved on to look at some of the specific principles on which a recovery approach is based, drawing on Anthony's (1993) seminal article and a research project. It is helpful to reflect on what these mean and how they can help service users move forward in their recovery, as often principles are presented as lists of positive virtues. Instead recovery represents a set of interlinked and consistent beliefs that represent valuable ways in which life might be lived in a rewarding manner.

In the chapters in Section 3 of this book we build further on this and look at models of recovery. If we are to effectively facilitate recovery with our service users, it is necessary for us to have a personal understanding of recovery, and have practised recovery on ourselves. We also look at how we communicate in a recovery-focused manner, before considering self-awareness, and then how we can use reflection and clinical supervision to develop ourselves as recovery-aware practitioners.

Section **2**

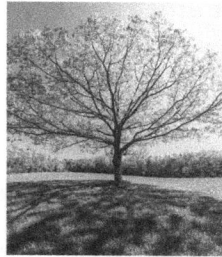

Using a recovery approach

3 Communication

Nick Wrycraft

Introduction

People are innately social beings, and thrive on interaction. Even the most self-sufficient person needs others. We are likely to struggle emotionally and psychologically in the absence of meaningful relationships and social contact. Communication is not something that we do just to impart information, it has an innate value in its own right. Many people with mental health issues have limited social networks, and may experience problems engaging with others or establishing and maintaining social relationships. This compounds the already detrimental effects of experiencing a mental health problem. It also leads to the absence of social support that many of us take for granted but which performs an important protective factor for mental health and well-being.

Communication is at the heart of therapeutic engagement and developing a genuine and human relationship with the service user is essential. Increasingly engagement with other current service users, or those who have experienced mental health issues is being recognized as a valuable therapeutic support. These networks can sustain long-term well-being and help prevent relapse.

The concept of recovery emphasizes the need for effective communication and collaboration as an essential part of the therapeutic process. In this chapter we discuss recovery-focused aspects of communication and the role it serves. We then look at styles of communication that emphasize the strengths of the service user, positive values and empowerment of the individual before considering the role of empathy.

In this chapter we will consider:

- What is communication?
- How we communicate in a recovery-focused manner.
- Communication and the role of empathy.

An understanding of communication – 'It's more than just about talking'

Communication serves a range of purposes. In one sense we communicate to impart and share information – messages are sent and received. But it

Figure 3.1 Simple communication – Imparting and receiving information

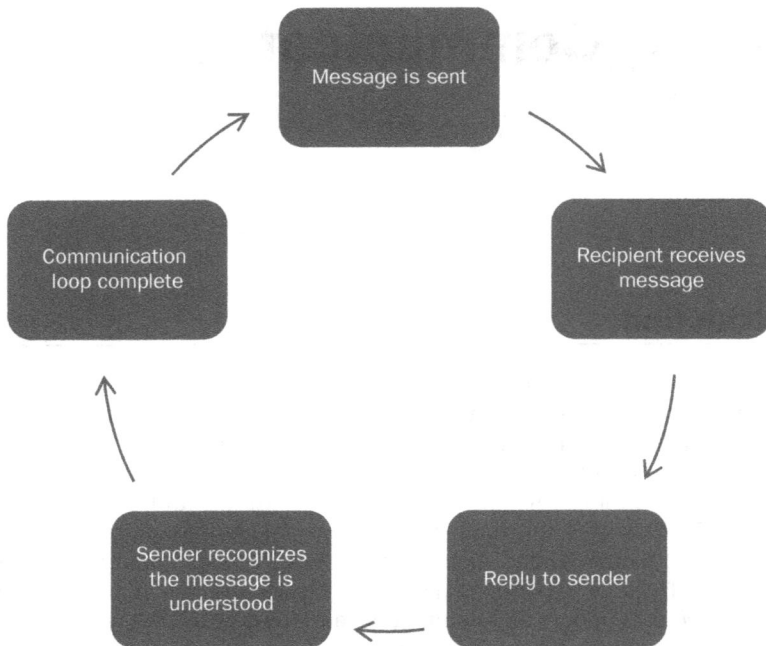

also needs to be two-way with both parties active in the process. The sender produces a message that is received and there is a response. From this the sender then understands whether their communication has been understood or not (see Figure 3.1).

An example is of me being lost and asking a passer-by for directions. If the person knows where my destination is and can tell me the route to my destination, and I repeat it back to them, then they know that I have understood them. Yet this is a simplistic notion of communication involving the imparting of facts and details. Communication with people experiencing mental and emotional distress is not just about exchanging facts but involves feelings and emotions, active listening and empathy, and the use of a range of verbal and nonverbal and interpersonal skills. When working in mental health settings we use our whole self, in a genuine and attentive manner that is wholly focused upon the service user with the intention of building genuine and trusting relationships (Williams, 2014).

In life when communicating we develop rules and understandings to establish mutual expectations and acceptable behaviour. Often this is a tacit and unspoken process, and we speak or behave in a way that seems to be right. Sometimes we might contemplate saying something, but are aware that the setting or context is not appropriate. This demonstrates a sense of self-awareness and orientation to our social situation. In some cases in practice, however, we may be working with service users whose ability to distinguish boundaries is impaired. Our role as a mental health nurse in accordance with the Nursing and Midwifery Council (NMC) Code (2015) may then mean that we have a duty to advocate for the service user. For example, I may be working with a service user whose mood is elevated and who is insistent on telling me something they feel is very important. The pace and rate of their speech may be extremely rapid and insistent, so that I cannot really follow what they are saying. I listen to them and do not display any outward impatience, but at a convenient pause in their delivery suggest they speak more slowly. In order to ensure the pace remains at a reasonable rate, and to help them keep the thread of what they are saying, I occasionally and discreetly break into their delivery and offer summaries. I might also state at the beginning how long I have for the conversation and stick to this time limit. In another example the service user may be experiencing psychosis and I may struggle to make sense of their speech content, or it may consist of disconnected ideas and comments. As opposed to questioning and interrogating them, it may be preferable to offer reassurance and to simply accept what they have said. This is different from colluding and pretending what they have said all makes sense. Instead offering reassurance respects the person's dignity and provides social inclusion where they may be acutely unwell.

As well as interaction, communication also allows us to express our beliefs and values through our culture. Respecting and valuing other cultures often take the form of a 'hands off' approach. We permit people of other cultures to practise their customs but remain at a respectful distance, with little real understanding of the meaning or value of these practices to the person. When we encounter people of other cultures, it is surely preferable to try to learn about the meaning of their beliefs and customs. In cultural expression and communication, we seek and provide acceptance, share affirmation and establish and reinforce a sense of belonging and social inclusion. Cultures share a sense of identity through common customs, for example, what we wear, celebrations, and rituals and way of life and belief (Wrycraft, 2015). All of these characteristics contribute towards cementing a sense of identity, but also support groups of individuals in establishing social cohesion or a sense of belonging.

A further purpose of communication is simply to share time and enjoy the company of other people. Social and leisure time is essential in terms of mental well-being, feeling able to relax, enjoying the company of other people and experiencing quality of life. Often we communicate to pass the time and simply to be with friends and people whose company helps us to feel better and good about ourselves.

There is a significant emphasis on technology and people communicating via social media within our society. Do you feel social media has a positive influence on society? On the one hand, it could be said that all communication is a good thing, and we are now more able than ever before to access and engage with other people. On the other hand, this often leads to us failing to engage with the people directly around us, and that many online friendships are little more than acquaintances.

Overall though it is easy to get carried away and give false prominence to a passing trend. People have an inherent need to communicate, and will always find a means to achieve this goal, and so our current preoccupation with technology could be seen to be more to do with this than an inherent interest in gadgets. While social media may feel omnipresent at the moment, trends change. If we were having this discussion in 10 years' time, we might not be talking about social media in the form that we currently know, but it is likely there will be another means by which we communicate. We might look back in astonishment at how we put up with straining our eyes looking at the small screens of our iPhones and iPads.

Yet even allowing for not being able to be in the same place as the other person, technology also serves as a means of therapeutic communication in mental health, and potentially even therapy (Cherry, 2017). In one study, taking part in virtual reality simulations reduced service users' paranoia (Medical Research Council, 2016), while there are numerous apps that can be used to help with an array of mental health issues (Kiume, 2013). These offer the advantage of being easy to use during our daily lives, and there is no need to attend appointments. They may also avoid the issue of labelling and stigma, as often these are available to everyone if they are inclined to look. Furthermore, telephone or online counselling is now easily available, convenient to access and fit into the busy lives people lead. Yet it is still most often the case that mental health nurses interact with service users through face-to-face communication. Interpersonal communication involves not only what we say, but also everything that accompanies it, including verbal utterances and sounds, facial expressions, body language and positioning. Understanding how we may use interpersonal communication well and reading and interpreting the communication of those with whom we interact are essential if we are to form and engage in genuine and positive therapeutic relationships and work effectively with service users.

Exercise

Make a list of all of the ways that you can think of in which we communicate directly with other people.

Compare your answers to the following list:

- verbal communication;
- verbal utterances, such as 'uh-huh' or 'mmm';
- facial gestures;
- facial expressions, such as smiling or frowning;
- body movements, such as a nod of the head, or a shrug of the shoulders;
- eye contact;
- touch, for example, a hand on the shoulder to demonstrate understanding.

Can you think of any other answers not already listed above?

Communication also occurs in terms of how we behave. For example, if I am extremely anxious about my interview for the pre-registration mental health nursing course, I may appear abrupt and preoccupied, and this will be apparent in addition to what I communicate. My body language may be stiff, and I may be less inclined to smile or be as friendly as usual. This will communicate how I feel about the situation, and inevitably influence how I conduct myself within the interview. Often people make allowances as it is understandable for a person to be nervous in an interview situation. However, it would be expected that the person can still cope and not be overcome by their nerves.

Communication is apparent through a number of different phenomena all happening at the same time and a collective response, reception and reaction between the parties involved. Often we 'read' this astonishing amount of information contained almost instinctively, and form instant impressions of the person's overall disposition, intention and meaning in a certain situation. Without the accompaniment of facial gestures and expressions and nonverbal communication it is so much harder to be able to ascertain people's meaning in communication, and recognize how they respond to what is being communicated. For example, have you ever had a phone conversation with someone you may even know well but the conversation is stilted and awkward? You interrupt each other and then both go silent waiting for the other to talk. Another example is that we might read the written transcript of a conversation between two people and form a conclusion as to how each participant feels and the nature of the exchange. Yet if we were to then see film footage of the same exchange, we might make a quite different interpretation of the encounter. This is because all of the other visual aspects of communication, such as facial expression and outward representation, add subtle but crucial inflections to verbal content that plays a vital role in determining what we mean, but also how what we are communicating is understood.

It is often said that first impressions count. Yet due to being such a natural and instantaneous process, it can be very hard to identify why we form impressions about other people so quickly. However, we all know when we are left with an uneasy feeling about someone, or the sense that there is something not quite right in what we are being told. Often this is due to contradictions in the message and the form in which it is delivered. For example, if I am delivering a presentation to an audience about confidence and assertiveness but clearly appear anxious even if I am attempting to place people at their ease, the inconsistency between the content of my message and the manner of it being imparted may leave people unconvinced. My audience may go away feeling dissatisfied with the presentation, but perhaps unsure as to why. Conversely, another person who is skilled in concealing their anxiety may deliver exactly the same presentation, but instead create a different and more positive impression within the audience. In most situations it is both easier and more straightforward to be consistent and honest about how we feel in relation to what we are doing. In the above example, if I were to remark, even just in passing about how anxious I am, this might change the atmosphere and transform how I feel, so I become more relaxed and find communicating easier. Yet at the same time my audience may become more receptive – or not, it depends; effective communication is reliant on numerous factors. But sometimes in mental health nursing, we may experience similar feelings of doubt, anxiety or even fear, but be obliged to reassure other people or portray confidence. If we refer back to Chapter 2, there may be a sense of dissonance between how we are obliged to act as a professional and principles of practice and the values we have as an individual. Often simply through experience we learn how to cope and manage challenging situations, but an important part of self-awareness is listening to ourselves and knowing how we make the change and where this feels comfortable or leaves personal conflicts and compromises.

Case Study 3.1   Lee

Within the last 48 hours Lee has been admitted to an open male adult acute unit. He has been in contact with the mental health services over the past 10 years as he was diagnosed with schizophrenia in his late teens. Lee is known to use illicit substances and has been admitted due to increasingly chaotic and disorganized behaviour at home and aggression towards his neighbours. He has been known to be violent towards people and in the past during previous admissions has assaulted members of staff. Although being an informal admission, Lee has made it clear that he resents being on the unit and has been talking loudly in the day room, making insulting comments to the nursing and catering staff and being aggressive towards other service users. There are concerns among the staff that his gradual deterioration in behaviour will lead to aggression towards either another service user or staff. George is the staff nurse in charge of the shift and is discussing what to do with the nursing team.

Q: How do you think a mental health nurse might respond?

Suggested answer: It might help for a member of staff to talk to Lee in a designated quiet room on the ward. In some cases, however, from a risk point of view, it might still be felt necessary for there to be two members of staff present. Yet the effect of two mental health nurses talking to one service user may interrupt the interpersonal dynamic and inhibit the flow and ease of the conversation. It may be plain to Lee that there are two members of staff due to concerns over the possibility of him becoming violent and lead to him becoming more hostile towards the ward team.

George as the nurse in charge felt he should speak to Lee. Another staff nurse discreetly waited in the corridor in case the situation should deteriorate George sat near the door and was visible from the window. Initially, Lee was angry and said he wanted to be discharged immediately otherwise there was no point talking. Instead, rather than disagree or contradict Lee, George patiently listened. He reflected back to Lee that he seemed agitated and understood why Lee might feel this way. During the conversation it emerged that before the admission Lee felt he was not coping with looking after his home or managing his money and self-care well and so in spite of being hostile to being on the ward, he seemed to understand the reason why he was there and how this might help. George told him that perhaps the admission might have come at a suitable time and discussed how he might use the opportunity to sort out some of the issues that he knew needed attending to and Lee agreed. In communicating with Lee, it is necessary to convey a relaxed manner and to listen to and consider his concerns. George was conscious of his own body language and remained seated, kept a relaxed posture, engaged in occasional eye contact and used a quiet tone of voice.

George tried to avoid 'hot' topics that he knew made Lee especially angry, such as it was felt that he needed to be on the unit at the present time. George also avoided themes of conversation that Lee might feel limited his choices. For example, instead of saying Lee needs to remain on the unit at the moment, George asked him what he hoped to achieve while on the ward. At the same time, however, George was vigilant of any increase in Lee's agitation, which might be evident in his body language, by, for example, sudden shifts in posture, animated gestures or preferring to stand up and walk around as opposed to sitting down and speaking. Where Lee seems to be getting agitated in mood or angry over a specific issue, George could respond by changing to another less contentious subject that he finds less confrontational. Or if Lee is standing up, asking him to sit down in a calm manner and enquiring if he is okay. It is not necessary to agree with all of what Lee says, but to be tactful. This approach will not be adopted all of the time, as recovery focuses on the service user taking responsibility. While there may be subjects that Lee may not like, these still need to be discussed, but can be tackled another time when he is more prepared. When he is likely to be aggressive if exposed to stressors, it makes sense to avoid topics he finds challenging.

George felt very anxious about talking to Lee even though he has been working in mental health nursing for many years. In spite of long experience and even if you have been in similar situations numerous times before, each experience is new and we all have feelings and emotions about those encounters. This is how it ought to be, so that the feelings that service users express are met with a genuine, humane and compassionate response. Yet George is aware of his strengths as a communicator and knows that he conveys a calm manner and is able to relate to people by listening to them. George still remained constructive and listened to what Lee had to say.

Communication is a skill we use constantly, and, as we have it, can easily go wrong and lead to misunderstandings; it is easy to become complacent. When working in mental health nursing we are often communicating with people we do not know well, or with people with whom we do not have a pre-existent rapport, so it helps to be clear and transparent, and honest in what we do and say. Crawford and Brown (2009) developed the Brief, Ordinary and Effective (BOE) Model, with numerous features but with the aim of keeping communication BOE. This approach emphasizes the need to express ourselves succinctly and clearly, though not abruptly, using clear and jargon-free language, and respecting others and different cultures while focusing on clinical practice and tangible outcomes. At the same time it is important that, while still being appropriate, not to be excessively formal but 'who we are'. Often service users feel disempowered in clinical settings as there is a power imbalance between the professional and the service user. Ensuring that we even out this imbalance wherever possible is necessary, and facilitating the service user to make decisions will help even up the relationship. It is also worthwhile taking into account issues the person may have with engaging in communication, such as low self-esteem, anxiety and being indecisive, and working to ensure that these issues do not impede the interaction.

The role of the mental health nurse in communicating with the service user is also therapeutic through facilitating communication. This may take the form of helping the service user develop an understanding of what they are experiencing and putting it into words. But also exploring what meaning they derive from events, and helping to identify a preferred and helpful response through identifying possible alternative choices of action. The intention of this is to promote empowerment and a sense of self-agency for the service user in promoting their recovery. In the next section of the chapter, we look at how we can work with service users to use communication to both practise and promote recovery.

Recovery-focused communication – How are you?

A frequent greeting made in passing or opening question for conversations is 'How are you?' Mostly this question is intended as a cursory enquiry, and the expected response is 'I'm fine.' The purpose is not to really ask how the person is, but is intended as a social device. In the same way when walking down the street if we see people we know, we often ask how they are, but, we do not slow down our pace in anticipation that they will say no more than simply 'I'm fine', or 'Okay.' Alternatively, referring to our unspoken rules of communication, if they were to actually say how they feel, or to tell you how much they are struggling at a difficult time in their life, this might seem embarrassing or socially awkward. Perhaps this tells us a lot about how we live our busy lives and the surface nature of the manner in which we interact with other people.

Yet when working in mental health nursing, asking the person 'How are you?' with the intention that they will tell us exactly how they feel is a commonplace expectation. It is important to be aware that it is an immense privilege for people to share their innermost thoughts, feelings and experiences with us in a way that is not the case in other social settings. This requires immense trust and courage. It may also feel unusual for the person to put into words the innermost emotions that they have perhaps never shared even with their closest friends, family or partner. Sometimes, however, sharing these feelings with another person who was previously unknown to them might be easier to do than with a family member.

In spite of the privilege of service users sharing their personal information, it is still the case that to be effective, communication ought to be spontaneous, and to feel comfortable. In this sense, even where sensitive or traumatic issues are being discussed, it is helpful to avoid using technical terminology unless absolutely necessary and avoid pathologizing behaviour also. For example, 'you feel like this because of . . .' explains behaviour. Instead, it is better to listen and understand, and for the exchange to be a conversation as opposed to a therapeutic encounter. Crawford and Brown (2009) suggest actively developing styles of therapeutic communication that are ordinary and straightforward. This avoids the use of jargon, terminology or complex ideas but instead allows us to engage transparently with the service user in helping them to bring about positive change and recovery.

Where people are experiencing dementia, for example, the ability to communicate can become compromised. The rate and nature of impairment also vary widely depending on the nature of the dementia. Often people experience difficulty in word finding, remembering what it was they began to say, remembering events or relevant information in a discussion, or understanding what someone else is saying. The person may also feel low in mood, agitated or anxious when engaged in communication as they are well aware of the difficulties. All of these factors can make communication even more difficult. This might appear to place significant obstacles in the way of effective communication, but, as we have established, communication is about more than imparting and receiving verbal information. Emotional and psychological aspects of communication can be conveyed in tone of voice, gesture, or timing, for example. People may feel embarrassed or ashamed at experiencing memory problems and immense frustration at finding it so hard to express themselves in ways that used to be so easy. Not focusing on problems, but seeking to overcome them in practical ways, can ease the process and reduce the impact of difficulties. We might simultaneously assess the person's communication difficulties and seek ways to overcome any limitations, using the responses of the person as a guide. For a person experiencing symptoms of dementia, then, we might interact as follows:

– When the person cannot find the word that they intended to say, avoid inter-rupting to say the right word as they may lose confidence, but instead indi-cate that we know what they mean and encourage them to carry on.
– Reassure the person by reminding them of what they began to say if they introduced a topic and then forgot what it was. Or perhaps offer a brief summary of the conversation so far to jog their memory or to provide some continuity to the conversation. This does not contradict the intervention immediately above as overall conversational themes are a shared factor, whereas the individual words we utter feel more personal. Being corrected over our choice of words feels more prescriptive than simply getting some guidance on where the conversation was going.
– Where the person has a memory lapse, and simply cannot remember what it was they were about to say and we cannot work out what it was, avoid asking a succession of questions or making a 'big thing' out of it, as this might increase the service user's awareness of their limitations.
– If the person cannot understand what you are saying, then try to explain another way, or unless it is important for them to understand, convey

acceptance that we might not be able to understand one another but can still communicate and that it is okay.

- Where the person struggles severely with verbal communication, always remember the value of nonverbal gestures, and enhance words with appropriate gestures and expressions of emotions to emphasize communication.
- While in many clinical areas touch is discouraged, when working with people with advanced cognitive impairment, touch may become a frequent form of therapeutic engagement, though should always be used sensitively and discreetly. For example, if I am guiding a service user along a corridor where there is a turn or change of direction they might not see and I am holding their arm to offer support, I might guide their arm gently in the direction we are going. Together with the shift in my posture as we walk, the person is likely to go with the cues offered and walk with me. Prompts of these kind often work where the service user requires support with self-care needs such as washing and dressing. This raises issues of consent. However, where the service user has high dependency needs, these will often have been discussed by the multidisciplinary team (MDT) and be considered in the care plan and documentation.

Q: In contrast, consider the case of another service user, Linda. She is picking up cushions that have been spread all over the floor in the day room of the adult inpatient unit, except there are no cushions. Linda has schizophrenia and is prone to hallucinations. Linda has asked you to help her and is busily engaged in the task but you can't see any cushions. Linda stops, looks at you and says: 'We don't want anyone to trip over them, aren't you going to help me?'

Would you:

a) help Linda by fetching a cone from the domestics' cupboard to block off the lounge until all of the cushions have been moved, and then help her as best you can;
b) say to Linda something like: 'Linda, I believe that you do, but I don't see any cushions so can't help you pick them up';
c) tell Linda she is hallucinating, and that there aren't any cushions.

A: We need to be honest with Linda and avoid colluding with her. So it is necessary to tactfully but honestly point out that we do not share her experience. At the same time it is necessary to point out that we believe she is having the experience. Therefore answer b. seems to be the most accurate.

Q: Could this undermine the therapeutic relationship?

A: The role of the mental health nurse is to advocate for the person. While this might be difficult, if handled sensitively, the service user will become aware that the mental health nurse offers honest responses, which is the basis of all functioning therapeutic relationships. Aspects such as consistency, perseverance, patience and reliability will all build trust and engagement with the service user. The techniques that are used will differ, depending on the specific circumstances. They form an important part of rapport building with the person and serve to establish an understanding on which to build therapeutic engagement. Engaging with the person in a manner that accommodates their needs or difficulties is often met with a sense of relief by the person and can facilitate commitment to the therapeutic relationship. In other words, the person will help us to help them. Careful observation and understanding therefore of the person's needs and accommodating this within our communication will help to nurture positive, productive and ultimately supportive therapeutic relationships.

Recovery also emphasizes hope and a positive disposition towards the future. In the case of the person with dementia, while they may not regain communication skills, it is still possible to experience meaningful interactions with others, and to feel valued and happy. Too often in clinical settings where we are under time pressures, interactions and giving attention to service users become restricted due to time limitations. Spending time developing rapport is essential to the development of the therapeutic relationship.

Within a supportive therapeutic relationship, the service user may feel more inclined to take positive risks, and make positive life changes. Often behaviours that are unhelpful to us become 'locked in' like default patterns. This is even more the case if we feel:

- A low sense of self-esteem, from the perspective of 'no one cares what I do anyway'.
- A lack of confidence to make a change and be able to follow it through.
- Low motivation and the energy to carry out the change.
- Feeling overwhelmed at the complexity of change.
- Even though other behaviours might offer other and perhaps better rewards 'I can't believe it, so will carry on how I am.'

Exercise

Q: Can you think of any activities that service users might attempt if feeling more supported?

Possible answers: Healthy behaviours that might be pursued include exercise and healthy eating, while unhealthy behaviours that might be changed include stopping smoking, giving up drinking alcohol and taking illicit drugs. Others include voluntary work, beginning an educational course, returning to work and taking up a new leisure interest. Or even visiting somewhere new, or going to a place of interest or event that the person might have always or long wanted to do but never felt confident enough to do or indeed that they were worthwhile pursuing.

Even small behavioural changes can lead to significant boosts in confidence and self-esteem, as well as a sense of the person taking control of their behaviour and doing something healthy. Other examples include stopping sugary drinks, choosing healthy snacks to sweets, and getting regular health checks or going to the dentist. On a more social level changes include varying long-established routines, for example, going food shopping somewhere new, visiting friends the person has not seen in a while or renewing contact with old friends.

Communicating with the whole person – the role of empathy

We can understand people better if we can appreciate their viewpoint. We might never share the same view, but very often we can understand why they see things how they do if we look at the world from their perspective. Empathy is often described as *standing in the other person's shoes*. Recognizing some of the factors and influences that lead to them seeing the world how they do, and making their present choices helps us see the person in context. This is helpful in allowing us to relate to them. Yet we can only arrive at such an understanding through spending time with the person and reflecting on the factors that are active within their life. We may expand our capacity for empathy by challenging our limitations, and those issues about which we have preconceptions.

Exercise

Think of a behaviour that you struggle to understand, and why you think this is. Next consider why people carry out this behaviour. There are two examples you might want to read as follows:

Example 1

- *Behaviour that I find hard to understand*: I struggle to understand how a person can harm themselves. I struggle to understand how it might feel to contemplate hurting myself with all of the possible detrimental physical consequences and long-term pain that might stem from that one incident.
- *Why people carry out this behaviour*: People carry out self-harm for many reasons, often to reduce high levels of emotional distress. As a result I may feel an alleviation of uncomfortable feelings. Pain also leads to the release of endorphins that create a pleasant sensation.
- I may self-harm because I believe that no one cares, and am trying to make my body dislikeable.
- People who have experienced abuse carry out self-harm, due to feelings of guilt or unwarranted self-revulsion for attracting the abuser. Or as a means

of trying to appear unattractive to the abuser to avoid experiencing abuse in the future.
- Within society there is a high awareness of body image, especially for younger people, and many struggle to live up to these perceived expectations. I may carry out self-harming behaviour because I feel I am falling short of this ideal.
- Often people feel that they lack power and control in their lives. Self-harm is generally carried out in secret, due to shame and embarrassment, and the not unreasonable concern that if known about, it may be stopped. Therefore, having control over the self-harming behaviour allows the person to have some power of this aspect of their life.

Example 2

- *Behaviour that I find hard to understand*: I do not understand why people drink, take drugs or gamble to the point that it dominates their life to the exclusion of all else, including financial hardship and loss of relationships. People have a choice, and so it seems illogical to continue to make the same unhelpful choices in the face of overwhelmingly negative outcomes.
- *Why people carry out this behaviour*:
- Alcohol especially is easily available and socially acceptable to use, yet easy to become dependent upon. The person may begin with casual use and gradually become caught in a pattern of repetitious behaviour that is hard to change.
- Behaviours that are more specialist, or even illegal have more closed and secretive networks through which people acquire and engage in the source of their dependence. Often people use drugs, for example, with their friends and peers. This serves to normalize behaviour, and makes change difficult, as in order to undergo the process of withdrawing from an addiction the person loses their friendship group, their lifestyle and support.
- Often people do not realize they have a dependency issue and may continue working, engaging in relationships and family life at the same time. The realization may only occur where there is a crisis, for example, financial issues, perhaps due to the addiction, or within relationships where partners, families or significant others lose patience with the person's behaviour, or it escalates to an intolerable level.

The act of caring is replete with thoughts and emotions, and good mental health nurses care, so it is necessary to recognize and acknowledge how this affects us. In some cases, we feel a particular sense of identification and connection with a service user. This might be because they are of a similar age or background to us, or have the same interests. Alternatively, they may remind us of a relative or friend, or their situation might remind us of something similar in our own life. At the same time, we can experience the reverse, and a sense of caution, insecurity or even dislike of a service user. Where either situation is the case, it is important to reflect upon how this affects our response to the service user. For example, are we being too pleasant and compensating for our dislike when engaging with the person we struggle to feel positive towards, or are we identifying too much with a service user to whom we feel a particular attachment? It is important to share how we feel in supervision with mentors and colleagues, so that we are practising honestly and responsibly. Therapeutic communication and interaction involve investing the self that includes not only cognitive aspects and the thinking part of us but also how we feel. Arguably, the two can never be disconnected, because how we think intimately affects how we feel and vice versa, and in mental health nursing the connection between the two needs to be closely integrated.

The outward appearance of emotion is not always an accurate indicator of what the person feels. For example, a person may feel extremely anxious and struggles with emotions that feel overwhelming, but hides them due to shame and embarrassment. Another person who is experiencing paranoia, while not displaying any suspicious body language or actions such as frequent checking and watchfulness, may stay awake all night due to their fears. Then there is the person who feels so low they want to end their life and does not disclose the extent of how they feel because they are concerned they will be admitted to an inpatient unit. The point is that when as mental health nurses we engage with the person and are casually assessing them, even the most traumatic issues may not be readily apparent. This does not mean that the service user is engaging in subterfuge or being evasive; it is simply that how we respond to our experiences and feelings can vary and take different forms, and as a mental health nurse it is necessary to get to know the individual. People do not always communicate what is happening to them, even where this is traumatic and highly significant. This does not mean that the person is being dishonest; it simply means that we are adept communicators but are also very good at coping and accommodating issues within our lives. Yet sometimes everyone needs help.

All communication is a fresh event and often we cannot predict our own responses. It is important that we listen to how we communicate with other people and reflect upon it afterwards, especially when an encounter has not gone how we might have expected, or leaves us feeling preoccupied or confused. When first meeting people or in an interview or tense situation, people can become stilted, awkward and more prone to communicating in ways that produce a response that we might not intend. It is important to take ownership of our style of communication. Bear in mind that there is no fixed right or wrong in these matters; this can be liberating, but also places an extra sense of responsibility on the mental health nurse as there is no single 'right answer'. While I might say something that I later feel was indiscreet, if placed in the same position again, would I say the same thing? Often we might regret the choice of words that we use, or feel anxious about the impression we might have given, but still feel that we have made an important point. We might do something slightly different next time, and feel that we have learned from the experience, but we can understand why we said what we did in the situation. When we feel that we get communication wrong, therefore, it is important to accept responsibility, understand why it happened, apologize to other people if needed, and forgive ourselves and commit to doing it differently in the future.

Conclusion

In this chapter we have talked about what communication is, how we can work in a recovery-focused manner, and how self-knowledge can enhance our skills. Due to being hard to define, elusive and something that we carry out almost instinctively, it is very difficult to honestly reflect on our communication. Often we deceive ourselves that we are better at it than we really are. Empathy is crucial in helping us to work effectively with service users. In this respect when learning in practice we are as much learning about ourselves and our own preconceptions as the service user's issues. When working in mental health nursing our main tool is ourselves and who we are. Gaining an honest understanding of our strength and areas and how we need to develop as communicators will help us improve our performance in practice and mean we relate even better to service users. This offers more beneficial therapeutic relationships and the prospect of real progress for service users. Continuing with this notion of working towards knowing ourselves better, in the next chapter we look at self-awareness.

4 Recovery and self-awareness

Nick Wrycraft

Introduction

In Chapters 1–3 we looked at an understanding of recovery and values before considering the principles of recovery, and then communication. Moving on from this, we now look at recovery and self-awareness. We begin this chapter by looking at how people with mental health issues are perceived. This is often subtle, yet highly damaging for people's recovery. As mental health practitioners, it is essential to promote and advocate positive views of service users. We then look at how mental health nurses can identify and resist stereotyping, and instead motivate and collaboratively support service users to achieve their goals and aspirations.

Embracing a recovery-focused approach that emphasizes openness and transparency, while adhering to professional boundaries, will help us to work with responsibility and integrity. In order to do this effectively, we need to look inside ourselves, and be aware of our own misconceptions. In developing as learners, however, we need to look at the motives that led us to work in mental health, as discussed in the exercise in Chapter 1. We need to reflect upon how we can use these as forces that exert a positive influence in our work. This takes courage, commitment, and a willingness to confront our own frailties and vulnerabilities. We also look at our own perceptions and self-awareness and think about how we can use these to contribute positively to our learning. Finally, we discuss setting some recovery goals for ourselves to realize our own potential and aspirations.

By the end of this chapter we will have:

- thought about the impact of misconceptions regarding mental health and stereotyping;
- considered what self-awareness is and how it can be applied to ourselves in our professional and personal life;
- set some recovery-focused goals to achieve our aspirations.

Misconceptions about mental health

Although progress has been made, society still often regards people with mental health issues negatively with suspicion, and in a way that is not the case with other serious health issues. This is disappointing, as providing mental health-care in the community is long established and we encounter people with mental health issues every day and in all social settings. There are numerous positive and very public role models of people who happen to have a mental health issue, yet we still do not have to go far to encounter ridicule, suspicion and hostility. Historically, people with mental health problems have frequently been regarded as part of a social sub-class alongside the poor and the economically and socially deprived. The vulnerability of this group of people is increased by the often unpredictable nature of society's response. At various times the mentally ill have been regarded with, on the one hand, pity and as victims, yet at others scapegoated and seen as responsible for all of the ills of society. Currently both views are apparent. For example, people who experience addiction or dependence whether to alcohol, substances, prescription drugs or gambling or those who self-harm or have a personality disorder are often regarded with scorn and seen almost as to blame for their issues. There is a view among many that the problems faced by these groups of people have been brought upon themselves.

While attitudes towards people who misuse substances, such as 'why should my taxes go on helping these people when they make a conscious decision to do it to themselves?', are never very far away, in contrast, people with dementia are often seen more empathically and with much greater understanding. The perception is that dementia is a devastating disease for which there is an absence of effective treatment, but also that often people with this illness have done nothing to deserve it. Mental health is an umbrella term that covers a wide range of very different problems with different causes, explanations and features. Arguably, neither of the above attitudes does much to empower the service user. Often people who misuse substances, self-harm or have a personality disorder bear the additionally disabling burden of self-loathing and loss of esteem. In the case of a person with dementia, they may be only too well aware of the sense of loss and pessimism that is often seen as accompanying this condition. In this chapter we look at how unhelpful misconceptions really are, but also how we might develop recovery-focused understandings and attitudes to promote a positive and proactive approach in our work with people with mental health issues.

Exercise

Step 1: On your own, or together with a friend, think of, and then write down all of the different terms used to describe a person who has a mental health issue. These can be formal or informal, slang references, those that are used casually, or even insults.

A sample list has not been provided as many of these words are insulting. You, on the other hand, can write down as many as you wish because at the end of the exercise you might want to tear up the piece of paper on which you have written the words and put it in the bin but keep your other notes.

Now count all of these words.

Step 2: Next think of another major health issue, and with your friend write down all of the terms by which it is described.

Once you have completed the task, count up the number of words that you listed and compare it with the total number you listed for mental health.

It is likely that there are far fewer terms used to describe the second health issue. Why do you think this is the case?

Step 3: Look at the terms you have listed for mental health, and on a new piece of paper write two headings of 'Offensive' and 'Non-offensive' and then group each word under one of the headings. Do not spend too long examining your thoughts or making decisions but instead work on the basis of what you already know, as the next part of the exercise will go into the *why*?

Step 4: When you have completed allocating all of the words, go through them again, and consider why you have chosen to categorize each word as 'Offensive' or 'Non-offensive'. This will take a bit longer, as you will need to think about your choice in each case, and also what each word means. In some cases you might need to look up the origins of the words as well, and this might add to your understanding of their meaning but also in some cases reinforce your choice to decide that the word is 'Offensive' or 'Non-offensive'.

- Did you find more words under the heading 'Offensive' than 'Non-offensive'?
- Do you feel that based on looking at these words that, overall, society has a negative view of mental health?

Step 5: Next, imagine that you are a person with a mental health diagnosis, and reading these words describing mental illness. How might you feel? Do you think that seeing the views of mental health represented by these words might influence how people feel about themselves?

If you were carrying out this exercise with a friend, discuss your perceptions of how the person with a mental health diagnosis might feel and whether this might influence their feelings.

Q: What have you learned from the above exercise?

A:

- that mental health is the subject of far more misconception than other major health problems;
- that some terms which appear to be innocent are laden with negative values, and that we need to be careful in the language that we use;
- people with mental health issues may feel the words used to describe them and their experiences to be deeply offensive;
- other, please add.

The words that we have considered above to describe mental health stem from, and represent, underlying concepts and ideas, and a frame of mind that views mental illness unfavourably. Examples include 'nutter', 'fruitcake' or 'loony' to name some that are older and milder but there are also phrases such as 'sandwich short of a picnic' that are designed to be almost witty, but is a cruel and withering (though often used) observation. It might be thought that in themselves these terms are harmless; however, for people who may already feel vulnerable and isolated, the effect can be highly damaging.

Some of the factors that contribute to society's view of mental health are summarized below:

- Many popular soap operas, TV series and films have had plotlines and characters that involve mental health issues. There have been some realistic portrayals, yet on other occasions, even in those that are renowned for their realism, this has not been well done, is misinformed, or the mental health issue has been exaggerated to increase the dramatic impact of the programme at the expense of portraying the true reality.
- Increasingly, sports stars and celebrities are admitting to experiencing mental health issues. This serves as a reminder that wealth, fame and status in itself can be stressful, and that we can never tell how a person really feels by what we see on the surface. Wealth and status, however, allow easy access to the best treatment and care that for many people lower down the social scale is not available. But celebrity accounts and experiences, while raising the profile of mental health, often do not represent the reality of ordinary people.
- The images of old asylums, and the associations of mental health with extreme and sometimes macabre crime are popular. There are popular myths about mental health that make good stories, whether true or not, and which endure within our cultural memory.
- Some mental health issues are particularly vulnerable to preconceptions, for example, personality disorder, substance misuse and self-harm. People experiencing these issues are often judged, held responsible or blamed for their problem.
- Mental health problems such as schizophrenia and psychosis are often regarded with fear due to occasional isolated and exceptional cases that are given undue emphasis in the media.
- There is still much debate and conflicting opinion over the causes of mental illness. As a result there are many views over the treatment for mental health problems.

Overall mental illness is much mythologized but often not well understood and frequently the subject of stereotypical perceptions and assumptions. Some of the above factors fascinate people, yet it is worth considering to what extent these perceptions reflect reality and are experienced as damaging to the self-perception of the individuals affected and their families, carers and significant others.

As a result of mistaken societal perceptions, many people with mental health issues feel disrespected, misunderstood and hurt at not being seen for who they really are. In many cases, a diagnosis such as schizophrenia or personality disorder can lead to individuals being treated with suspicion or fear and experiencing social exclusion and discrimination.

Exercise

What springs to mind when you think of:

- someone with schizophrenia;
- someone who is depressed;
- someone who has a personality disorder.

1 Did you have a specific gender for the person?
2 Were they of a particular age?
3 What specific features did that person have?
4 Now think about why you might identify a particular mental health issue with someone of a certain gender, age and with certain features.
5 Why is this the case?

It is human nature to compare previous situations or highlight resemblances with those we encounter next, and so we all engage in stereotyping. In this way we can learn from experience and anticipate what to do when confronted with a similar situation in the future. However, stereotyping can mean that we fail to see the specific differences between situations. This can lead to the person feeling that they are not seen for who they really are, that they are grouped alongside others, often those with unflattering traits, not all of which they may share, and that their unique perspective is not recognized. Yet we all make stereotypical assumptions, even over the smallest of things.

Exercise

Think of yourself in terms of features that might be used to define you. For example:

- gender;
- age;
- where you are from: country/county/town;
- height;
- weight;
- interests;
- school/college you went to;
- do you have brothers/sisters? If so, how many?

While providing some details that are specific, this information is just a thumbnail sketch and does not really say anything about you as a person. From this vague overview, we cannot possibly know who you are, in terms of your disposition, personality, preferences, likes and dislikes. Someone may have the same characteristics as you, but be completely different as a person. From these general characteristics, we are not able to know about your motivation, sense of hope, or what you wish to do and aspire to in the future. In stereotyping we take these rudimentary features about a person and make other assumptions about the person as well. To be judged by general characteristics that you share with many others can feel impersonal, highly offensive and that you are not seen as an individual.

Exercise

1 Have you ever felt stereotyped in terms of any of the above information, or in another way?
2 If so, how did this feel?
3 How might this learning inform how you will work with service users to avoid the negative effects of stereotyping?

People with mental health issues often report the consequences of social exclusion to be worse than the symptoms of the illness itself. Frequently, people not only experience negative perceptions from society but also may feel shame, self-loathing and an impact on their self-esteem as a consequence of mental illness. Sometimes even the mental health services provided to support people with mental health needs contribute to this experience. It is worth bearing in mind that we all make assumptions but to avoid damaging effects on service users, we need to work hard to always see the individual in front of us. Consistent with recovery-based practice, everyone should be treated as a unique individual. In Chapter 3 we talked about every interaction being a new instance of communication, as well as the importance of listening to the person and regarding everyone as an individual.

For example, in practice, consider how often you hear the same or similar situations being described. However, for that person their experience is still unique and attendant with that are a whole set of responses and emotions that may or may not be similar to those of others. It is important that we respond in a manner that reflects and is congruent to the service user's emotion and not become blasé or complacent. While we may have seen many service users in a distressed situation, if we become casual in how we respond, this will be evident to the person, who will then not feel listened to or acknowledged. Instead we might consider why the person is feeling how they are, and how we might help them to explore and understand their emotion.

Within recovery, helping the service user to process what happens to them and fit it within the context of their life is extremely important if the person is to make progress and move forward. However, it is also worth remembering that healthcare professionals learn from the experience as well. We need to consider the effect of our interactions with service users in terms of how it fits with what we believed that we knew before, and how this may challenge what we now feel and think.

Q: How might we begin conversations with service users that avoid making assumptions?

A:
- In our general approach making a point of actively involving the person in all conversations, and while not testing out absolutely everything, at the same time not making unreasonable assumptions. For example, 'you said to my colleague last time that you didn't mind sitting down any time and talking about your care plan. Am just asking, is it okay if we talk about it today?' As opposed to automatically assuming the person is willing to discuss their care with you.
- Be prepared to be corrected, and receptive to the person's preferences, choices and perceptions.
- Checking names and titles: Does the person want to be called the name that is on their notes, or something else? It may be spelt incorrectly, or there are not enough characters on the form to permit the full name to be entered. Some people prefer to be addressed more formally as Mr or Mrs as opposed to their first name.
- Checking facts: Is what we understand about the person correct? While it sometimes helps if we already know about the person's situation not to ask them to go through the whole story again, often and especially in relation to a significant event, people want to present their own version, even if this is the same as what we already know. From a recovery perspective, hearing this and listening acknowledges the person and their perspective and will help in developing the therapeutic relationship.
- Because a person appears to adopt a certain lifestyle does not mean that they necessarily embrace everything that commonly goes with it. For example, following a particular religion does not mean that the person adheres to every custom or action.
- In a similar manner, people may not behave consistently with the beliefs they profess. Instead they may interpret and have an idiosyncratic way of life that we need to have explained to us in order to understand.

It is naïve to believe that we can ever view everyone without preconceptions. So it is important that instead we can recognize where this occurs, and how we might alter our behaviour. Often mistaken perceptions stem from limited knowledge or experience with a certain group within society. This may be in terms of age, gender and sexuality, race and ethnicity, spirituality or socio-economic group. In the absence of direct knowledge, we may make assumptions that may be influenced by the media and what is known more anecdotally about the group to which this person belongs. While some groups within society are quite clearly defined in terms of their features and membership, others are much less clear. Some groups that might seem very identifiable are more subtle. For example, a male who wears feminine clothes or a female who chooses to dress in a style deemed to be masculine may be regarded as being gay, yet this is by no means necessarily the case. Why people choose their clothes can be for many reasons and communicate many different things. Also what is deemed to be masculine or feminine clothing is a matter of opinion, therefore, we need to be sure of the basis on which we form conclusions about people. Yet at the same time people may provide subtle or discreet indications about who they are and to which groups they belong without wishing to make overt declarations as to their identity. Consequently, we need to tread a careful line between overestimating what we can know about other people, yet at the same time failing to see what is plainly right in front of us. This is a skill that can be developed with practice and experience, but requires continual self-awareness and the capacity to always be open to learning and practising in accordance with the NMC Code (2015) in continuously focusing on promoting and advocating for the person's mental health and well-being.

In practice, therefore, we need to reflect upon and challenge our assumptions. For example:

- Is the person whose family says 'he is lazy – he's always like that' really lazy, or depressed or low in motivation and mood? We may have encountered someone else in the past whose situation was similar and who we thought was also lazy, but does it mean this is also the case in this instance?
- Overestimating insignificant or random details. For example, because I choose to dress in a way others feel is unkempt, am I neglecting myself? Or because I wear a lot of black or dark coloured clothing, am I depressed or low in mood?
- Assuming that we all have the same priorities. For example, a person may be living with cancer yet may feel this is not their priority. In some cases people avoid, deny or minimize the problem; they may lack knowledge, or they may simply feel this is not the most important issue on which they wish to focus.
- Assuming that the trigger for a relapse is the same as the last one. For example, is the person low in mood because it is wintertime as they also relapsed at the same time last year, or is it just a coincidence?
- Assuming that a person can never change unhelpful behaviours. For example, many people with addictive behaviours will express a wish to change at numerous points in their life. It is important for us as their supporters to always believe that change is possible, because one day it might just happen.
- Assuming that a person will just be prone to repeated episodes of depression and anxiety. For example, while it is true that the more episodes of depression a person experiences, the more likely a further one is to occur, there may be other criteria by which we can measure success, such as if a person stays well for longer than they have managed for a few years before. Or if

for a period of time the person has a period of extraordinarily good quality of life, even though this may be sandwiched by episodes of illness, then perhaps this still represents a success.

- Assuming that someone does not have the potential to achieve their dreams or wishes. If the mental health nurse does not believe the service user can make a change, then their support will not be as effective, and their interest and regard for the person not genuine. For example, a service user sets a goal that is impossible. As opposed to tactfully but positively trying to negotiate a more realistic objective, the mental health nurse simply goes along with the person's wishes and lets them fail. While the motive might have been to let the service user learn by experience, this is a cruel way for them to find out. Although recovery empowers and prioritizes the service user taking control of their care, the mental health nurse's role is still to facilitate and represent an honest sounding board for the service user's goals.

Of course, in some circumstances, all of the above assumptions may be true. What is important, however, is how we use and apply our knowledge, so that it is selective, based upon careful judgement and is focused on the person in front of us. Guesswork has no place here. As we have established in Chapters 1–3, self-reflection and the work we carry out upon ourselves as developing practitioners are essential in ensuring that we are able to engage with service users in a manner that allows us to be receptive to their viewpoint. But we also must be able to understand their situation as clearly as possible, and help in a way the service user finds useful. These seem like simple and quite obvious precepts, but as we have seen in the discussion so far all sorts of barriers can get in the way.

Often the circumstances of the situation lead to an assumption that the person has a mental health issue as the only way of explaining behaviours. For instance, consider a person who was admitted to A&E after drinking a large amount of alcohol and taking substances and overdosing on prescribed medication. This is an often repeated scenario, and depending on various factors the decisions made and outcomes vary. However, the risk-averse nature of specialist mental health services can lead to assumptions being made; for example, in the above case the person was making a deliberate attempt to end their life. Instead it helps to ask what might seem like obvious questions where we are left with doubt or gaps in the story, for example, 'What were your thoughts when you took the overdose?' The answer may elicit a range of other responses, such as:

- 'I felt desperate and just wanted to stop feeling so bad.'
- 'I just don't know. One minute I was in crisis the next I was taking the pills.'
- 'It seemed to happen in slow motion, there I was just taking these pills and it felt like someone was else was doing it as though I were watching a film.'

All of the above provide different possibilities for the therapeutic response to the person. Our scope for working with the person would be much more limited if we make the assumption that their overdose was a deliberate attempt to end their life, without seeking their explanation or viewpoint. If we proceeded from this perspective, there is the possibility that the person may feel that their actions were misunderstood and experience distress at the kind of assumptions being made regarding their intentions. Furthermore, exploring the event serves a therapeutic process. It can help the person frame the situation within their own mind, and where necessary recollect and perhaps gain a sense of control over a situation in which they felt overwhelmed, or as though reality were happening outside of them. Yet, as you can appreciate, sometimes there are behaviours or sets of circumstances for which there are several similar but all different explanations. For the person the difference is crucial and if we are to form an effective therapeutic rapport and working alliance with them, we need to gain as accurate an understanding of their situation as possible.

In the next section we look at how we explore our own feelings. Often these are elusive and difficult to define. However, being open and willing to explore these feelings, initially with ourselves, and then perhaps with others, will allow us to develop and work more effectively with service users.

Working with ourselves

In ancient Greece at the famous oracle at the temple of Apollo at Delphi, inscribed above the entrance was the phrase 'Know thyself.' It has been rumoured that this is only part of the inscription. Yet the significance of this message being at the entrance of the temple is that before we can learn about anything else, we need to understand ourselves first. To be able to effectively use knowledge, we need to be aware of our own starting point, and only once we begin to know ourselves, can we make sense of anything else. Yet we can only gain self-awareness through 'working with ourselves' and this involves honestly examining our assumptions and preconceptions and who we are (Freshwater, 2002; Healy and McSharry, 2011).

Sometimes the ideas and beliefs that we hold most emphatically and resist challenging are those that we most need to re-evaluate, or even let go of completely. This can be hard, and it is very often tempting to just hold on to our views and opinions anyway. Even where they no longer work for us, or prove to be unhelpful, familiarity and habit can make them feel comfortable. Yet we need to understand that preconceptions may cause real harm and contribute to genuine misery and distress on the part of service users. While the NMC Code (2015) requires that we promote the interests of the service users, and that we strive to challenge ourselves, it is important to be aware of and to recognize the transition of our ideas in terms of how we develop and progress. Through reflection, we can become more aware of our views and how they influence our thinking and attitudes. If we are to support service users to the best of our capabilities, then it is necessary to realize where our attitudes exert both a positive and negative influence throughout the personal and professional transitions that occur during our training as a mental health nurse.

It can be difficult to adapt to a new role. Often in making this transition, certain aspects of our personality become more pronounced. For example, if I am prone to perfectionism, I may become even more pedantic, while if I see myself as an academic I may mention theory more in my conversations with my peers. However, it is worth considering the effect that we have upon others. For example, my perfectionism may be seen as excessive and an unnecessary attention to detail, and that it is all I care about at the expense of other more service user-focused issues, while my emphasis on theory may make others feel inadequate if they are not as confident on this particular aspect. Often the impact we have on others is not deliberate, or not intended, so as peers and colleagues it may help to be patient and understanding with fellow students when making changes to the fundamental ways in which we engage with service users and each other. Yet at the same time, there is an obligation to provide honest, though tactful and constructive feedback if we are to make progress. Giving and receiving feedback on our style and manner of communication and how we 'come across' are essential in learning (Esmiol and Partridge, 2014), and in mental health nursing.

There are several other pointers to remember about work:

- Mistakes are a part of learning. Often the best learners are not those who make the least mistakes, but those who learn the most from them.
- Be open to feedback, and actively seek it from others as often as you can. This not only demonstrates transparency, but that you want to make the best of all learning opportunities.
- See the feedback in context. If it pertains to a formal assignment and relates to specific marking criteria, this is different from carrying out a peer-led exercise with fellow students that is not formally assessed. This does not mean though that some learning is 'better' than others. Sometimes we can learn a lot when not being formally assessed, as we are more relaxed and behaving as our natural selves.
- All learning is of value, and we can learn from any situation.
- Do you find some comments or characteristics used repeatedly to describe you in feedback given by different people? Do you agree with these descriptions and can you see what they mean?

As a result of feedback it is important to set or re-evaluate learning goals and priorities. At any time as a student mental health nurse, there needs to be personal goals that we are working towards in addition to the formal academic or practice assessments on the course. These may be in relation to aspects of practice, or concerning personal attributes. Examples include:

- becoming better at asking open questions in assessments of service users in practice;
- ensuring my lack of confidence does not show when talking to service users who might, for example, be much older and have more life experience;

- feeling more comfortable and knowing when to ask significant questions, such as 'why do you act on thoughts to carry out self-harm?';
- being able to contribute in multidisciplinary team (MDT) meetings;
- feeling able to be assertive when talking to my mentor and explaining how my outcomes might be met.

Often these will be consistent goals to which you return time and again during training. In Chapters 1 and 2 we encouraged you to consider how your personal values relate to the principles of the profession of mental health nursing, and reflecting on this will provide a solid basis for your development. It is also important to keep track of your progress. Often we look at our former selves when we begin to reflect and feel embarrassed at the views and opinions we expressed. But in order to be able to trace your emerging identity, it will help to keep a record. This may be through:

- keeping a journal or diary, whether this is a hard copy version, or
- written records of discussions with your mentors in your practice document, such as action plans designed to develop and advance your learning in the clinical setting. Or your reflections based on feedback from written assignments earlier in the course to develop your understanding of theory.
- regular clinical supervision, either as part of a group in the practice setting, or with fellow students;
- meetings for tutorials and discussion with mentors or tutors.

It is also necessary at certain times to stop and review your progress and consider what has changed, how you have developed, and in what ways.

Q: How will you know if self-reflection makes a difference?

A:
- Reviewing reflective accounts and identifying the changes in your approach, and development in your knowledge and attitudes, over time.
- Feedback from peers, colleagues, lecturers, friends and family.
- Feedback from service users.
- Generally feeling satisfied and fulfilled at work and in your personal life and being aware of meeting challenges and demands.
- Able to clearly identify new goals for your learning and development, as this never stops.

Consistent with the philosophy of recovery we are all individuals, and as discussed at the end of Chapter 1, the motivation that causes us all to want to work in mental health nursing is different and wide-ranging. It is important that we understand how this influences our approach and the ways in which we are likely to be affected. As a result we can become better at managing our own emotions, understanding our own needs, knowing what we gain from mental health nursing, how this influences our work with service users and maintaining a healthy balance in our lives. Yet most importantly we will be aware of what our skills are, what we give and how we can facilitate recovery for service users. Often this is significant in how we attribute personal meaning and feel about our work with service users and our attitude towards mental health. Yet this is also a powerful force and drive in sustaining us through our career, and determining the direction it takes. As the following case studies illustrate, there is no perfect pathway leading into mental health nursing.

Case Study 4.1 Jackie

Jackie is a mature student mental health nurse, and experienced physical and psychological abuse over a prolonged period as a child. Following treatment for her issues as an adult, Jackie entered mental health nursing after a career where she ran her own business. Jackie describes the reason for the change in career as simply that mental health had been in the news, and one day she thought 'why don't I go and help people for a living?' Jackie is remarkably unaffected by her traumatic experiences. She says she feels surprised and lucky that it does not affect her more. At the same time though she feels a sense of guilt when she sees other people who have been so dramatically impacted by their experiences. When going onto placement, Jackie was concerned that she might feel a heightened sense of emotion or connection when working with survivors of abuse that might make it difficult for her to cope. Outwardly, Jackie is very confident and capable and tends to cope with things alone, which might mask difficulties or lead to these suddenly becoming significant issues due to her coping for a long while without disclosing that she is experiencing difficulties. However, Jackie meets regularly with her personal tutor to discuss her progress, and feels that she has been well supported by mentors on placement to the extent that she could disclose any issues that she might have.

Case Study 4.2 Simon

Simon's older brother James had a drug and alcohol problem that lasted from his late teens to his early thirties. Simon's mother went through a lot of distress, and he can vividly remember when he was younger seeing her very often upset and worried over James. Simon wanted to help, but felt powerless. James was eventually able to move on, and has been drug- and alcohol-free for the last five years. Sadly, James and Simon's mum died of cancer a couple of years ago while in her fifties. When on placement on an open acute unit, Simon was working with a young man who was admitted to the ward as a result of drug and alcohol misuse over a prolonged period.

Simon realized that he felt angry towards the service user. He was careful not to show this, and to treat him as fairly and the same as anyone else, and in fact the service user seemed to enjoy a good therapeutic rapport with Simon. However, Simon felt like a fraud and that his real feelings, although concealed, undermined the sense of transparency in the therapeutic rapport. He discussed this situation with his mentor, and Simon realized he felt the same way towards the service user as he felt towards his brother. He felt the same sense of powerlessness in being unable to help the man change his behaviour as he had when he had seen his mum upset at James's behaviour.

Furthermore, on reflection, Simon realized that he believed there was a connection between his mother's cancer and her worry over James. As a result Simon had always blamed James for his mother's illness, and felt angry towards him. This realization has helped Simon move forward in his own life, and he feels contributed towards his development as a student mental health nurse, as he felt less resentment towards the service user. As a further outcome from his reflection, Simon decided to learn more about addictions and substance misuse, and why it might be hard for people to bring about behaviour change.

Case Study 4.3 Lia

Lia experienced anxiety and depression from when she was 15 years old. She limited what she ate and drank and began engaging in self-harming behaviour. Eventually she was admitted to a child and adolescent mental health unit. She did not gain her predicted grades due to experiencing these difficulties at the same time as her GCSEs. Lia is now 23 and after gaining employment in a number of different jobs has found working as a carer in mental health to be something enjoyable and rewarding. She topped up her qualifications so that she could meet the university entry requirements. In spite of being aware that she is bright, Lia expresses feelings of inadequacy, and is daunted at the prospect of going to university, saying that only the subject of mental health and the thought of becoming a qualified mental health nurse have stopped her withdrawing and not taking up the place. Lia discussed her concerns with her course leader and personal tutor. They advised her that she should look for the objective evidence before jumping to conclusions as to her capabilities and progress, and that by meeting the entry requirements for the course Lia is as eligible as anyone else to study mental health nursing. Lia has completed year 1 of the course, and passed all of her theory assignments and practice placements. She is aware that she has high expectations of herself and her performance, and still often has doubts and cannot believe she is a year 2 mental health nursing student. However, Lia actively works at monitoring her thinking so she can detect when she may be excessively hard on herself.

All of the above examples represent realistic perspectives of student mental health nurses. While in many cases there are aspects of our performance that we need to work on, it is important that we do not regard these as *mistakes*, as this can lead to us making negative appraisals of our own capabilities. Often the attributes that lead to unhelpful thinking styles also have the potential to produce positive outcomes. For example, attention to detail and a methodical approach can lead to perfectionism that can stop you doing things because of concerns at not getting everything exactly right. Yet this same attribute is useful if you are engaged in work that requires precision and being exact.

Exercise

Consider your understanding of mental health before beginning the nursing course. Was this drawn from:

- experience of family members with mental health issues?
- experience of friends and acquaintances with mental health issues?
- personal experience of mental distress?
- being at school, or working with people with mental health issues, either as co-workers, or encountering people with mental health issues through work?

It is necessary to use our understanding in a way that promotes positive growth and adaptation. This comes from more than simply the desire to help or from identifying with the person. Consider the factor(s) that you have identified above and how your training as a mental health nurse corresponds to that motivation. You may well have more than one reason and, if so, the list does not necessarily need to be in order of priority. Next consider how you as a student mental health nurse will translate that source of motivation into a goal that prioritizes the recovery of service users (see Table 4.1). Think about what might help you in achieving your recovery-focused goal. Finally, consider what would constitute the achievement of your recovery-focused goal.

Table 4.1 is an example of a recovery-focused personal goal. It is worth bearing in mind that it is best not to make these too specific in relation to a particular mental health issue, or link them to the role of the mental health nurse; for example, by referring to the NMC Code (2015). Also remember that recovery is not exclusively about moving forward, and so achieving the goal might not occur in one act or even the service user's mental health seeming to improve. If the person feels that they have made progress, then this represents a step forward. Instead, recovery recognizes the fluctuating nature of mental health, an ongoing process which means that recovery happens afresh every single day for us all. A recovery goal, therefore, within the role of the mental health nurse, may be continuing to work with people who are acutely unwell and in crisis.

Table 4.1 Recovery goals

Motivation for becoming a mental health nurse	Goal	Resources	Achievement
Mum's depression and anxiety, and feeling I couldn't help when she got really low, and it felt as though the illness took her entirely away from us when she was like that	To help people break through the grip of something like depression and support them in challenging low mood	• To learn more about the many mental health problems that function like depression • To consider and help to better develop services and support carers and families of people with mental health issues • To look into psychological therapies that might be suitable for people with depression • To look into the function of medication for depression	• To be with the person when they are really low in mood, and persevering when they are at a low point and to reflect on that • To collaborate with the person on their care and recovery plan

Conclusion

In this chapter we have discussed a number of issues that may strike a personal chord and make you think. Working as a mental health nurse involves working with your feelings and your whole self in order to therapeutically promote the mental health of others. In life no one is gifted with all of the answers and we all have our own issues to bear. Anyone who thinks they do not is simply deluded and perhaps lacks the humility and self-awareness that might qualify them to work as a mental health nurse. Developing a positive and open sense of ourselves that cares for our own needs in a compassionate way is the first step towards becoming a good advocate for others. So before considering caring for others, it is important to be aware of our own needs and how these can be met. From seeing and feeling this success, we can move forward in the confidence that recovery works for us and so can work for others.

It is important that we realize we are all on a path towards recovery. Training to be a mental health nurse means that if we recommend recovery to service users, we ought to undertake it ourselves. Developing self-awareness is a lifelong commitment and hard work but pays dividends. Being aware of how we communicate is important. We can all think of people who are skilled and adept communicators but those who are poor communicators perhaps more readily spring to mind because problems with communication are more apparent than when the process goes smoothly. Through practising in a self-aware manner and applying the principles of recovery in our interactions with service users, we can facilitate our own learning. It is also worth being aware of the need to be humble, to always be willing to learn about ourselves, and further develop our own growing perception of what recovery means for us.

5 Reflective practice, clinical supervision and learning from experience

Allen Senivassen

Introduction

This chapter looks at practical approaches to promoting reflection in working with service users towards their recovery. It builds upon the discussion so far, from considering our values and principles, how we communicate and the importance of self-awareness. This chapter addresses the following points:

- Why reflection can be difficult, and the rationale for reflection as a mode of learning in practice.
- How to use Rolfe's (2001) reflective model, and keeping a journal as a means to aid reflection.
- Clinical supervision as a platform for reflection and the role of journal clubs in contributing to evidence-based practice.

By the end of this chapter the reader will have considered:

- a rationale for engaging in reflective practice;
- how to apply a model of reflection to practice;
- the benefits of reflection within a structured clinical supervision framework including group supervision;
- how journal clubs can advance evidence-based and reflective practice.

Reflection is a way of learning to develop professional practice, and can help us assess the way we think, feel about and carry out our work. Through reflection we challenge the basis of our beliefs, assumptions, values and principles (Wrycraft, 2015). When reflecting we consider aspects of our practice to which we would not normally give much thought or attention (Bond and Holland, 2010).

It helps us become more aware of ourselves and others and reconcile ourselves with the outcome of events in practice. Through reflection we also explore alternative courses of action that might have been taken. Yet reflection is not just about thinking, but in order to be meaningful it needs to generate changes and outcomes in practice (Wrycraft, 2015).

Why is reflection so difficult?

Experience provides a wealth of learning opportunities. We can take full advantage of these by turning our experiences into positive learning through reflection. There is an abundance of literature on reflection and reflective practice (Johns, 2013), and professional bodies such as the Nursing and Midwifery Council (NMC) expect practitioners to demonstrate reflective practice in their professional revalidation (NMC, 2015). However, reflection is not a feature of the natural pattern of work for most mental health nurses. Many nursing students also freely admit that they do not reflect on a regular basis, but may do so when compelled to, for example, on the care of one or two clients for the requirements of an assignment, or for the completion of their practice document. It seems, therefore, that reflection is neglected, and the full potential of what it can offer is being missed.

Q: Why do many students not engage in reflection?

A: Below is a list of comments from students who find it difficult to reflect:

- Not really understanding how to do it or whether we are doing it properly.
- We only do it to complete the practice document, or at the end of the placement.
- Mentors do not model reflection in their own practice due to heavy caseloads, or the culture in practice not supporting reflection.
- Too tired at the end of the shift to reflect on practice.
- Feeling bombarded with enforced reflection in coursework, assignments and practice documents.
- We reflect in university, but seem to go over the same point(s).
- It is often used inappropriately to criticize our mentors.
- The relevance of reflection to practice is not clear.
- Did you think of any others not on the list?

Bearing in mind these reasons, it is understandable that some students do not regularly reflect on practice.

In the current climate of staff shortages and heavy caseloads, the culture in the workplace is often not conducive to putting aside time for reflection. Qualified mental health nurses may recognize the value of reflection, but the NMC's (2015) requirement to keep a reflective portfolio for revalidation purposes can also make it appear to be an additional pressure and burden. Therefore reflection is not being carried out for the correct reasons, which sadly undermines the point.

Exercise

Having considered the practical difficulties and barriers, can you make a case for why practitioners and students should make reflective practice a reality?

There are good reasons why we, as healthcare professionals, should engage in reflection:

- We are constantly exposed to new experiences without being fully aware of their real value, but which might be helpful for us to learn from and from which to derive new knowledge and understanding. These experiences could be a vital source of learning, if only we were to stop and think.
- When reflecting we pay attention to ourselves and notice our thoughts, emotions, beliefs and values. In attending to how we feel about our work, and in challenging our own beliefs and feelings, we learn to become more empathic, positive and person-centred and recovery-focused in our therapeutic approach. As Boud et al. (1985) argue, through reflection we turn our experience into valuable learning.
- Through reflection we discover other ways of working to produce better outcomes for service users and their families. Reflecting on any practice experience, whether good or bad, is useful. But paying attention to a positive experience is more likely to reinforce positive practice. As Drucker (2011) explains, if you reflect on an effective intervention, this can turn it into an even more effective intervention in future.
- Working with people with mental health problems can be emotionally challenging, and to handle these demands safely, we must promote our own mental health and well-being. Through engaging in reflection and clinical supervision, we become more able to recognize the effects of emotions on our well-being, and become more resilient.
- Through reflection we become better at using theoretical knowledge to make sense of service users' situations and needs, develop more effective interventions and, in turn, establish knowledge for practice that we can transfer to other situations. This explains why the NMC (2015) requires us to demonstrate reflective practice in our professional revalidation.
- As students and practitioners we enter the profession to make a difference to the lives of service users. Supporting service users in reaching their full health potential is very rewarding personally and professionally. In turn, this leads to higher self-esteem, job satisfaction and creates a cycle of excellence.

- Through reflection our self-awareness grows as we evaluate and challenge our personal beliefs and feelings. We gradually make adjustments in ourselves to respond more positively to different situations (Wrycraft, 2015). Consequently, we become better colleagues to our peers, and more effective as autonomous practitioners. A reflective practitioner will often display an aura of inner confidence, compassion and optimism, which, in turn, instils hope in service users, and can reinforce recovery.

Using Rolfe's (2001) reflective model to facilitate reflection in recovery work

There are a number of different reflective learning models. These include:

- Bond and Holland (2010);
- Johns (2013);
- Kolb (1984);
- Rolfe et al. (2011).

Some are more elaborate than others, but essentially they share common themes and elements that provide a structure for reflection. When deciding on a reflective model, consider which one you find appeals to your way of thinking, and you find easy to use (Wrycraft, 2015). However, the depth of our reflection is not as a result of the chosen model but the way in which it is used. Rolfe's (2001) model depicted in Figure 5.1 was developed from Borton's (1970) model and has been chosen for its simplicity.

Central to Rolfe's learning cycle are three key stages, of 'What?', 'So what?' and 'Now what?' These are briefly explained, and then demonstrated by being applied to a particular case.

- The reflective cycle starts with the 'What?' stage that consists of describing the situation, relevant issues, problems and consequences. It also involves looking at feelings, and the responses of others involved in the situation and

Figure 5.1 Rolfe's three stages of the reflective cycle
Source: Rolfe (2001).

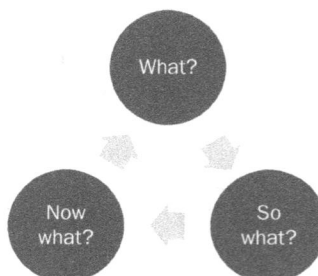

looking back at the experience and your emotions. This is best carried out soon after the experience, when all the information is still fresh in your mind.

- In the 'So what?' stage we examine our emotions and analyse the situation to become more self-aware. We explore the interventions used to decide what works and what does not work. In the 'So what?' stage, the aim is to find out what was happening from a more objective stance. You can begin to understand the perspectives of the various people involved in the situation, and make sense of why people have behaved or responded in the way they did. Looking back at yourself involves examining your thoughts and feelings, and how you performed. As a caring person you may be overcritical of yourself and exaggerate your weaknesses. It is wise to take a balanced view by giving adequate attention to your strengths as well as the areas requiring development. Developing emotional skills such as self-awareness and self-acceptance helps us remain calm in adverse situations (Bond and Holland, 2010) and work with sensitivity, empathy and compassion with service users in challenging situations.

- The 'Now what?' stage focuses on what needs to change in the future and what needs to be done differently to improve our practice. Having recognized in the earlier stage of reflection that our knowledge and skills need to develop in certain areas, we now devise an action plan. For example, if you recognize that more exposure to clients with different mental health problems is required to enhance confidence in practice, you may seek the support of your mentor to gain this experience.

To demonstrate how Rolfe's (2001) model can be applied in practice, the following example takes the reader through the three stages of the model using reflection on service user Joe's case by Carole, who is a student nurse, starting with the 'What?' stage of reflection.

Case Study 5.1   Rolfe's model applied by a student nurse

'What?' stage of Rolfe's model

'As a second-year student in a community placement, I went with my mentor Mary, a community psychiatric nurse with many years' experience, to visit Joe at home. This is a regular fortnightly visit to support Joe and his parents. Joe is in his late twenties, and has been a service user for the past 10 years. He has bipolar disorder, and has been feeling low lately. He lives with his parents who are in their sixties. My mentor seems to get on well with both Joe and his parents. They explained that he has become withdrawn recently and is not attending the day centre. Apparently, this is the usual pattern of events when Joe is relapsing and his parents are concerned that he receive more intensive help urgently. I sat next to Joe in the lounge. He was listening to the conversation but avoiding eye contact and being involved in the conversation. I tried to talk to Joe but he hardly acknowledged my attempts that frustrated me, as I thought

I could be of help to him. After a week of university study on recovery, I had many useful ideas for helping Joe. I felt disappointed I had not connected with him but also wondered if he resented what his parents were telling Mary.

At the end of our short visit I got the impression that Mary was not overly concerned, but she reassured the family that she would speak to the psychiatrist to arrange a home visit. In speaking with Mary afterwards she was aware of the complex dynamics and maintaining different but equally supportive relationships with both Joe but also his parents.'

Case Study 5.1   Rolfe's model applied by a student nurse (*continued*)

'So what?' stage of Rolfe's model

'I turned the focus of my reflection on my feelings during the home visit at Joe's flat. Mary, my mentor, had prepared me for the visit before we arrived. She explained the relationship between Joe and his parents, and the purpose of our visit, which is to support all of them. By the time we entered their flat I felt as if I knew the family based on the information I had received. Comparing this experience with a previous visit to a different client with another practitioner, Mary made me feel much more comfortable by the way she introduced me as a student colleague. She invited me to contribute to the conversation. I learned from Mary that the brief social interaction at the beginning of a visit creates a relaxed atmosphere for subsequent engagement. Yet at the same time she was engaging with both Joe and his parents, though on this occasion more with his parents than Joe, which on reflection surprised me as I was focusing more on engaging with Joe.'

The above extract shows Carole is reflecting on how supporting the service user in the context of their family involves supporting all of them, as opposed to just supporting the service user, and that sometimes other family members may be the central focus of attention.

Case Study 5.1   Rolfe's model applied by a student nurse (*continued*)

'Now what?' stage of Rolfe's model

'I am keen to become competent like my mentor Mary, and I know it will take me some time to achieve this level of competency. I checked with Mary whether her approach works with all of the families and service users living with carers and significant others on her caseload. Mary responded that it depends on the relationships and understanding how they work. In our discussion I realized that Mary is an experienced practitioner and used to working in the community with service users and their families and carers.

I as a second year student was just looking to connect with Joe. Mary took the lead with the family. I am not sure I would feel at ease and confident doing that at the moment but plan to work on taking a more active role when making visits in the community in future placements.'

Exercise

Select a client from your practice placement to reflect on and work through the stages of Rolfe's (2001) model. It is better to choose a client in whose care you have participated. This is because reflecting on an experience in which you have been involved tends to increase emotional connection and competency (Bond and Holland, 2010).

Examples of cases that students have used from their practice for reflection include:

- listening to a service user who self-harms;
- engaging with a service user who is contemplating suicide;
- responding to a service user who is traumatized by voices in their head;
- having a conversation with a service user with a history of aggressive behaviour;
- working with a service user who does not want to engage;
- accompanying a service user with agoraphobia to a shopping centre;
- motivating a service user who is in despair and has lost interest in self-care;
- working with a service user within the context of a complex family relationship;
- working with a detained service user who refuses to take prescribed medication for their mental health;
- experiencing conflict within the team;
- safeguarding issue relating to a vulnerable service user;
- working with a recovering service user who wants an immediate discharge into the community, but is at risk of relapse if the discharge is rushed.

Reflection on action and reflection in action

So far our discussion on reflection using Rolfe's (2001) model has concerned after an event has taken place. This is referred to as 'reflection *on* action' (Schön, 2008). Another example of reflection on action is when the clinical team meet to discuss and debrief after an incident, for example, on a ward after a service user has attempted suicide. The aim is for the team to support each other, analyse whether the suicidal behaviour could have been prevented, and to explore new ways of working to protect the service user.

Reflection can, however, also take place during the event, and is called 'reflection *in* action' (Schön, 2008). Although this may not be as deep as reflection on action, it can be of immense value, for example, in the case of a service user who appears to become more anxious as she talks to a student about her discharge home. The student reflects at the time on what is triggering the servce user's anxiety, and what can be done to alleviate it. This brief reflection in action helps the student to realize that she is out of her depth and this lack of confidence may be fuelling the service user's anxiety. Consequently, the student opts to bring the conversation to a gentle close, and reassures the service user that she will arrange for her care co-ordinator to see her.

Reflective journals

Reflection on practice is an activity that many practitioners undertake on their own during the course of their work. It can also take place, however, through a conversation with a mentor, colleague, fellow student or critical friend. Critical friends are our peers or colleagues who, while looking out for our interests and regarding us positively, will actively consider what more we might have done. Being open to feedback from a critical friend relies on mutual trust, and commitment to learning. The benefit of this feedback is to access a different perspective, and to reveal opportunities for learning and developing practice. To aid reflection, however, it is also recommended to keep a reflective journal.

A reflective journal facilitates deeper reflection through allowing you to write down your experience of an event, describing it and then analysing your thoughts, feelings and actions. Writing down your experience may reveal new and different aspects to the experience. For example, you may write about the experience of working with a particular service user in their home. You may then find yourself gaining greater understanding of their family context, relationships with other people, belief system about recovery, and what motivates or hinders their progress. As you continue writing, gaps in your knowledge, for example, about your service user's condition and your own intervention skills, may become apparent that need to be addressed. The initial writing down of an experience may start when you are in practice during a break, or soon after the shift ends. Using Rolfe's (2001) model, we can write the description of the experience according to the 'What?' stage while the facts are still fresh in your mind. Then at the end of the shift either at work or later on that day we can then proceed with the further stages of reflection.

You might use your written reflections in the journal in discussions with your mentor. This will make meetings more productive for both parties. Students will gain a deeper understanding of practice from different perspectives through discussing their written reflections with their mentor, while mentors, through understanding the way the student perceives practice in the written account, will appreciate the student's level of understanding and learning needs and be able to identify new and developmental points of learning for the student. The reflective journal is personal and confidential to each student, and you decide which reflective material you want to discuss at meetings with your mentor.

Reflection and clinical supervision in practice

The relationship and difference between reflection and clinical supervision are simple but significant. Reflection is carried out alone and is the focused and deliberate contemplation of specific instances or situations from practice, while clinical supervision involves a supervisor and supervisee, who also consider examples from practice. Yet in supervision, the supervisor or mentor helps the supervisee or student to develop new understandings and meaning from practice. It is this interpersonal aspect that represents a crucial additional dimension to the process. In contrast, in reflection the learning depends on the individual's ability to be self-aware, objective and challenge their own knowledge in generating new perspectives. This does not mean that reflection cannot be as productive as supervision. Only that supervision offers more opportunity for different perspectives. The supervisor is usually a more experienced practitioner and aids the reflective process by asking appropriate questions surrounding a client case or a clinical issue presented by the supervisee.

Exercise

Have you received supervision from your mentor or personal tutor or a critical colleague friend?

What has changed for you as a result of this supervision?

If your supervision was well facilitated, you would have experienced some of the benefits identified by Proctor (2008), whereby effective clinical supervision performs three interrelated functions (see Figure 5.2).

Figure 5.2 Proctor's model of clinical supervision
Source: Proctor (2008).

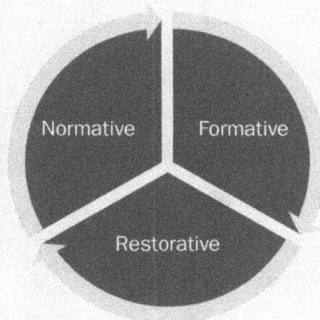

These are:

- *Normative*: The supervisee is helped to examine whether the level or standard of care expected by your placement setting and by the professional body is met and, if not, how the quality of care could be improved to meet the expected standard. Effective clinical supervision is empowering to supervisees, practitioners and students, and promotes reflective practice.

- *Formative*: The formative function focuses on enabling the supervisee to learn about oneself, and in developing new skills and knowledge from supervision. The supervisor helps the supervisee to recognize their contribution to the situation, and enables them to explore how they could extend their knowledge and skills further.
- *Restorative*: The supervisor ensures the supervisee feels supported and energized when discussing the case on which the discussion is focused, particularly if it was a stressful one. It can be cathartic for the supervisee to share feelings and difficulties about the case with a supervisor who understands and has empathy.

Clinical supervision can be as an individual, or in a group. As students you may have experienced group supervision in the classroom where each of you discusses individual examples. You may find more benefit from group supervision where your peers in addition to the group supervisor will bring different perspectives and further options to consider. One study found that students value group supervision when it has been well facilitated. They felt enlightened by the discussion and the feedback from their peers and the facilitator (Ashmore et al., 2012), while effective clinical supervisors have been identified as possessing a range of interpersonal, communication and competency-based skills (Skinner and Wrycraft, 2014). Group supervision is also preferred by management as it is less costly.

Exercise

As a student have you had any experience of group supervision?

What was your experience of the supervision like?

How has it changed your practice?

Earlier we used Rolfe's model to guide how an individual practitioner can undertake reflection of a client's case on their own. This model can also be used in group clinical supervision. Hawkins and Shohet (2012) suggest a structured framework for reflection in group clinical supervision that enables us to fully appreciate the wide range of different perspectives that are active within supervision. They identify four key aspects of practice for reflection and

Figure 5.3 Hawkins and Shohet's four aspects of clinical supervision
Source: Hawkins and Shohet (2012).

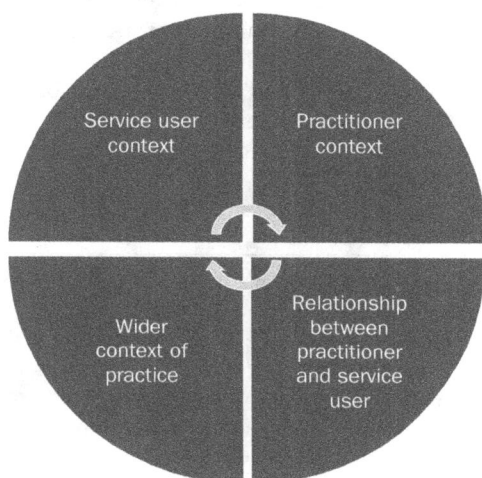

supervision, which have been adapted slightly for the context of client recovery in mental health settings. The four aspects (see Figure 5.3) relate to:

- the practitioner context;
- the relationship between the practitioner and the service user;
- the wider context of practice;
- the service user context.

The group supervision process starts with the supervisor setting the scene, clarifying expectations and agreeing the ground rules. The number of cases presented in each session depends on the size of the group, and the length of time it takes to discuss each case. Typical supervision group sizes vary from between 3–8 people (Hawkins and Shohet, 2012). Some groups begin with each supervisee briefly summarizing a case of their own, before deciding on one case to discuss in depth. The presenter describes the case for 3–5 minutes, and the supervisor and other group members tease out more information to build a comprehensive understanding of the service user's needs and interventions (Hawkins and Shohet, 2012). The group then builds a theoretical explanation of the situation, and discusses a range of options for intervention and likely outcomes. Finally the presenter, who knows more about the case, will consider which option or solution from those suggested is likely to produce the best outcome. To demonstrate these aspects we will apply them to the example discussed earlier in this chapter of the service user Joe and student mental health nurse Carole, who presented the case to her classroom group supervision facilitated by their personal tutor.

The service user context

The group considered the service user's needs and explanations for how these arise, including the causes and contributing factors. It is important to consider how the service user feels. The whole group then participated in thinking about how the service user feels and about possible explanations for their actions. The aim of the in-depth discussion is for the supervisee to develop a sound understanding of the case, before deciding which interventions may best suit the service user.

Exercise

Imagine you take the service user's case you selected in the earlier exercise to a classroom student supervision group. The setting is relaxed and your peers are keen to learn about the service user. What type of information do you think they might want to know? Here you are stepping into the shoes of your colleagues and asking yourself questions from their perspective. It is challenging, but can be a very worthwhile exercise, bringing issues to your attention about the service user that you had not previously considered.

Carole presented the details of Joe's case followed by gentle questions from her peers to enable them to understand the perspective of Joe and other significant people such as his parents and friends. Questions asked by the other students in the group included the frequency of Joe's relapses, what caused them, how Joe perceived his current situation, and what would have helped in his recovery. Through sensitive enquiry from the group Carole discovered that there could have been some conflict between Joe and his family regarding his recovery goals, and the means of meeting these. For Joe, recovery meant feeling good in himself, being able to concentrate on watching current affairs on TV and playing games on the computer. His parents, however, saw his recovery in terms of his attending the day centre regularly, and being more outgoing.

This discussion prompted one group member who had recently read about recovery to offer a theoretical explanation and refer to the relevant literature. Internal recovery is the feeling of self-esteem and inner well-being experienced by the client, while external recovery refers to how the service user relates to life and phenomena outside of themselves. It appears that for the family external recovery was more important. In the case of options for intervention, the group saw both perspectives of recovery as being conducive to Joe's well-being but that Joe should be at the centre of decision making in his recovery. The group also suggested that as an intervention the family could be helped in a sensitive way to understand the importance for Joe to make decisions and choices regarding priorities for his recovery (see Chapter 8 on families, carers and significant others).

As the discussion proceeded, another group member enquired whether stigma and discrimination were impacting on Joe. This student suggested that Joe's reluctance to attend the day centre may have been a sign that he felt safer in his own home, and was concerned at feeling different to other people. Carole acknowledged that the debilitating effects of stigma and discrimination did not seem to have been given due consideration in Joe's care, and she would discuss this with her mentor.

The practitioner context

The aim of group supervision is to help the supervisee to:

- feel supported in their practice;
- develop greater awareness of their strengths;
- become aware of their personal and professional values, skills and knowledge guiding practice, and to develop these to a higher level;
- recognize potential areas for development in order to become a more effective practitioner.

We are often not focusing on ourselves when engaging with service users (Bond and Holland, 2010). While we ought not to be exclusively focused upon ourselves, reflection allows us to develop greater self-awareness. As we consider practice, we recognize how our feelings, thinking and behaviour affect how we engage with service users and how we may develop our skills.

Exercise

Ask yourself the questions you anticipate your fellow students/peers might ask in group supervision. For example, they may want to find out about your thoughts and feelings and the skills used when you were with the service user. Or they may want to help you identify your positive attributes, and recognize the areas you need to develop to become more competent.

During discussion of Joe's case, Carole found out that she had a strong sense of hope that had developed after she recovered from a major illness in childhood. She felt she could use this positive trait effectively in her development in working with service users.

In terms of areas for self-development, through group clinical supervision, Carole became aware of the source of her frustration during the visit to Joe's home. She believed that Joe should be at the centre of the recovery plan, and yet his parents were allowed to take the lead. She felt the mentor could have done more to advocate on behalf of Joe and put him at the centre of decision making. Upon further reflection on comments from her peers, Carole acknowledged that the parents were acting in Joe's best interests rather than their own.

They had witnessed the pattern of his illness over many years, and how his condition deteriorated rapidly and disrupted the whole family.

Carole arrived at the conclusion that Joe and his parents did not have conflicting intentions but were working towards similar recovery goals. It was understandable that his parents sought access to help early when they felt his mental health was deterioraitng. As a result of this reflection, Carole was aware of having revised her stance towards Joe's parents, and their role in his recovery. There was also a similar shift in other group participants. It was interesting to see how this came about following a contribution from one mature student in the group who had a sick child. The latter explained that professionals sometimes find it difficult to comprehend the role of the family as full-time carers, handling the emotional and physical traumas of mental illness on a daily basis often without professional intervention. She argued that the family's role in care planning should be reappraised in each situation. The supervision not only helped Carole but also helped other peers in the group to develop a more informed understanding of the role of the family in being carers (see Chapter 8 on working with families, carers and significant others).

From the group discussion, it also emerged that Carole was annoyed with Joe because he did not respond when she tried to speak to him. Managing frustration with service users who take a long time to respond to questions was also an issue for other students. This provoked further discussion and an exploration of possible interventions.

One solution came from a student who mentioned that just sitting relaxed and being with the client is a positive, caring and compassionate intervention even if only few words are exchanged. The group concluded that we need to reflect on the criteria by which we judge the success of interventions and that we need to go at a pace that is appropriate for each individual's recovery.

Carole went back to her mentor to find out more about Joe's history. It transpired that Joe had an episode of mania with disturbed behaviour that led to a compulsory inpatient admission two years previously. Joe had hated the hospital admission because he felt his freedom was taken away and the staff did not treat him like a human being. Subsequently, an 'advance statement' was put in place consenting for his parents to make decisions on his behalf if he becomes unwell to avoid inpatient admission unless absolutely necessary. Knowledge surrounding advance statements and other terms was picked up in the journal club discussed further below.

The relationship between the practitioner and the service user

The relationship between the practitioner and the service user is perceived as the third aspect of clinical supervision by Hawkins and Shohet (2012). The quality of this relationship will often shape the nature of the service user's collaborative engagement in their recovery. The aim of reflecting on this relationship is to discover:

- whether it is based on mutual trust and respect;
- to what extent there is a power balance in decision making between the practitioner and the service user;

- how external factors are affecting this relationship;
- if experiences and emotions from previous relationships on the part of either the practitioner or the service user may be interfering in the current relationship;
- how the relationship could be enhanced to help the service user's recovery.

The relationship between the healthcare practitioner and service user is often fraught with difficulties, and could be a source of stress to both parties. If the service user feels unable to trust and confide in the mental health nurse, or compelled to accept treatment, they may disengage from the services. Developing a therapeutic relationship with the service user takes time, and practitioners with large caseloads may not be able to work as collaboratively as they might wish. However, the service user may understand and accommodate these difficulties if collaborated with and included in the process.

More difficult to deal with is emotional baggage from previous relationships that both practitioner and service user may bring. Emotions from previous relationships are often played out in current interactions, usually without either party being fully conscious of them. For example, we may treat a service user with greater affection because they remind us of someone else we know and like. If, however, we have had a traumatic relationship with someone in the past who resembles the service user, this may hinder the relationship without us being aware of it. Such countertransference of emotions by the mental health nurse may occur from time to time, and can be counterproductive in the service user's recovery. Similarly, transference may occur. For example, the service user may seem detached or aggressive towards the mental health nurse if they have had negative experiences with other practitioners or authority elsewhere. Clinical group supervision offers a good medium to enable us to recognize transference and countertransference in our relationships with service users.

Exercise

With regard to the case you selected for group supervision, can you imagine what types of questions your colleagues will ask you in order to understand your relationship with the client? Alternatively, you can focus on Joe's case and think of questions that you would like to ask Carole in order for you both to understand her relationship with Joe.

In the group supervision, Carole was asked by one of her peers whether the situation with Joe reminded her of any other situation she has experienced before. She recognized that Joe's case appeared similar on the surface to that of her own cousin whose mother was quite controlling over her grown-up children. To some extent she felt her aunt should have backed away, and that the children should have spoken up more. As the reflection progressed Carole became aware that her cousin's situation was different to that of Joe's, and that they were both unique in their own right. Carole noted that to develop healthy and trusting relationships with other people, she would need to contain and avoid feelings experienced in other relationships spilling over into new ones in practice. Other students also recognized that their relationships with certain clients might have been affected by previous experiences in a similar way, and reflecting on Joe's case helped them understand and take stock of their own emotional interpersonal issues. A key concern for the students was how to work collaboratively with clients who mistrust professionals which, as discussed below, will be the subject of a future presentation at the journal club.

The wider context: organizational and professional

Reflecting on care relating to an individual service user helps us consider how the profession and organization in which we work have an impact on how we deliver care. The aim of reflection here is to:

- Identify which key policies from our Trust or healthcare organization are directly implicated in the care of the selected service user, for example, is there a safeguarding issue for consideration? Does the lone working policy help or hinder your work with a particular service user?
- Examine how our professional body, the NMC, determines our professional consideration for the client, for example, are we providing care based on the best available evidence? What does best available evidence mean when caring for someone with specific needs? How do the '4Ps' (**P**rioritize people, **P**ractise effectively, **P**reserve safety, and **P**romote professionalism and trust) of the NMC Code (2015) apply to us when working with a service user and their family?
- Recognize whether there are resource implications related to the care of a service user that need to be highlighted, for example, can other disciplines be invited to contribute to an individual's care package?
- Apply appropriate guidance, for example, from the National Institute for Health and Care Excellence (NICE) to care delivery.
- Explore how the recent Mental Health Taskforce Report on *The Five Year Forward View for Mental Health for NHS England* (2016) will affect nurses' recovery work in future.
- Draw on the policies of local health providers and professional bodies to provide the best care possible for our clients. Do the policies raise dilemmas for our professional practice and how can we reconcile these dilemmas?

Exercise

If you were a colleague in Carole's group supervision, what questions would you ask Carole to help you both understand the impact of guidance and policy on Joe's case? Alternatively, refer to your own client case and reflect on which policies and guidance would apply.

In relation to Joe's situation, a number of questions were raised by the students, including these two key questions:

- How can nurses meet the 4Ps of the NMC Code (2015) in the face of increasing client caseloads?
- What are a crisis plan, an advance statement and an advance decision and how do they work in practice for a client like Joe?

The students in the group supervision identified that their mentors have to complete a large amount of paperwork, and this applied in Joe's case. Also, the students expected to witness more high-quality therapeutic engagement by the practitioners, such as social and psychological interventions. Instead they often witnessed frequent meetings with clients to monitor their condition and review medication, with little focus other than to ensure Joe was keeping to the prescribed regime. It transpired through discussion that staff were offering a safe service, but not necessarily the most recovery-focused approach. The students were not sure whether staff were using the best available evidence to inform their practice, and commented that these staff often appeared drained by routine work. They acknowledged that they needed to continue with the group clinical supervision to 'inoculate against burn out', as one student put it, and to build resilience in order to be able to maintain compassionate care. They recognized that the group would need to use more creative strategies to be aware of developments and best practice once they qualify.

The journal club

So far we have seen how evidence-based practice can be enhanced through reflection and clinical supervision. Yet a number of issues can arise that require exploration through further reading and research. With this in mind I suggest the development of a journal club in each practice setting. Journal clubs aid reflection and this idea was borne out of a series of discussions I had with participants attending clinical supervision workshops in various Trusts in the east of England between 2012 and 2016. The journal club is gaining interest among practitioners in various settings (Senivassen, 2016) as a way to augment reflective thinking, keep abreast of contemporary literature, research and policies, and to develop practice that is based on the 'best available evidence and best experience' (NMC, 2015).

How does the journal club work?

The club usually meets on a monthly basis, for approximately one and half hours, with a different person volunteering each time to present a recently published article that has direct relevance to challenges in the care setting. A summary is presented of the article followed by a facilitated discussion.

Finally, the group identifies key issues and learning arising from the presentation and outcomes to implement in practice.

The next session starts with an update on progress since the last meeting before another paper is presented. The journal club adopts the same principles as an action learning set with the aim of bringing evidence-based care into practice. An action learning set consists of a small group of people who define the challenges in the workplace and systematically set out to address them through discussion, the development of action plans, implementation of these and then evaluation.

The whole process of the journal club starts with the clinical team identifying the challenges in their clinical areas of practice, and using evidence-based literature for informed discussion, followed by actions by practitioners to improve care. Subsequent feedback on actions carried out between journal club sessions ensures staff consistently improve their practice as a result of the journal club.

Carole attended the journal club in her practice setting, and a colleague presented a paper on 'advance statements, advance decision and advance directives' by Jankovic et al. (2010), which was followed by a practice-based group discussion.

Why is a journal club valuable in practice?

- It takes reflection to a higher level. As we reflect on practice, we recognize gaps in our knowledge, values and skills. The journal club can help to address these deficits.
- The club enables practitioners and students to search for the best available evidence and to share and apply them to resolve challenges in practice. The whole team is kept in the loop of excellence.
- It engages everyone in the team, boosts morale and transforms practice quicker than when one individual attends a course or reviews a guidance or research paper on their own.
- The club stimulates a dynamic learning culture in practice and drives high standards of care for patients. At a time when funding for courses is scarce, the journal club offers an effective way of propagating knowledge among clinical teams.
- It helps mental health nurses complete their professional revalidation.
- The journal club directly links theory to the reality of the practice area.
- Practice is underpinned by shared best evidence.
- It is rewarding and enhances job satisfaction.

Exercise

Imagine you want to set up a journal club in your practice area, or for your group at university. How will you go about setting one up?

Impact of the journal club

The journal club is beginning to have some impact in practice settings in a local Trust where it has been implemented as evidenced by the comments from a practitioner and a student in a mental health recovery unit.

A practitioner commented:

> The journal club has benefited the ward by aiding continuous personal and professional development of the staff team. Our recent article on 'Dealing with borderline personality disorder' highlighted areas of development and improvement around care planning and mindfulness. As a result of this, mindfulness is now our next topic, due to us identifying a deficit in our practice. This evidence-based discussion in our journal club has added to our practice and knowledge of each other (via debate) and of how to care for service users.

While a student commented:

> I did not realize this level of discussion takes place in practice. The journal club is new to me. The discussion has given me hope that more can be achieved with challenging service users through different ways of working, and not just providing custodial care. I am excited with this development; the discussion has helped me to understand the theory for the way staff provide care . . .

Conclusion

Although engagement in reflection and clinical supervision is disappointingly low, increasingly students are recognizing not only the value but also the necessity of developing self-awareness. The perception of reflection is also not helped by associations with practice documents, outcomes and assignments, and being seen as complicated and difficult. Instead, reflection ought to be something that is accessible and convenient for mental health nurses to access. It also needs to be carried out routinely in practice if we are to make full use of the learning opportunities available.

This chapter has shown how a student can learn to use reflection through applying a model, and how this process can be aided by a reflective journal and taking part in a journal club. The more closely reflection links with and provides outcomes directly related to practice, the more beneficial it is proven to be. It is hoped that through using these mechanisms repeatedly through their training, and then seeing positive outcomes as a result of reflection and clinical supervision, current students will become the reflective mentors of the future.

6 The service user perspective

Melanie Cotter

Introduction

Unless we work with the service user clearly in mind, then we risk providing care that does not meet their needs or support their priorities. This chapter offers a perspective on what service users feel they need. It may seem unusual but often the attitudes of the mental health providers have been experienced by service users as discriminatory and harmful. Institutional discrimination is caused by prevailing negative attitudes within large groups of staff, such that the values of the organization become negative towards those whom we ought to be serving.

In this chapter the examples on which we focus are of service users with a diagnosis of borderline personality disorder (BPD). However, there are passing trends in the identification of mental health problems. In the past other mental health issues were regarded with the same concern as BPD is today, while in the future we can substitute still other mental health issues that are yet to be named. The process of developing diagnostic categories through clustering together shared and identifiable features is of debatable value in mental health. This is because these attributes are invariably undesirable and deeply damaging to society and the individual. This is even more concentrated with the current reductions in funding meaning services are harder to access and in consequence only service users with the most acute and debilitating issues are assessed as being eligible to receive care. Such diagnosis-led views run counter to the philosophy of recovery.

The impact of receiving a diagnosis is likely to have a significant impact on the person's self-concept, and views of their life. In this chapter we look at this aspect of the mental health nurse's role, and invite you to reflect upon the impact of this on your professional values for practice. We also look at how negative attitudes can detrimentally affect the therapeutic relationship between the mental health nurse and service user and impact upon care. Particular attention will be paid to people with BPD. Direct quotes from service users are frequently used and we end with two case studies. The purpose of this is to promote the use of the service user's own words and explanations for situations. This places prominence on the service user's perspective and demonstrates active listening in the most effective manner. We also consider how we might better support mental health nurses in developing more positive and less discriminatory attitudes towards people with mental health issues. In this chapter we will discuss:

- an appreciation of the service user perspective in practice;
- the effects of receiving a diagnosis, stigma and how discrimination of certain mental health conditions undermines a recovery-based approach;
- how mental health nurses can be supported to better deal with challenging situations and behaviours in practice.

What do service users want for their recovery?

The views of service users are often not sought or considered in their care. This is possibly due to the circumstances in which a person is admitted, for example, where there is an inpatient admission, there may be a crisis meaning that there is limited opportunity to sit down with the person to discuss their wishes. This can, however, lead us to make a range of assumptions about how the person feels and what they might want from their recovery. Some examples of what service users have said about their needs follows.

> I wanted to have hope, and I wanted to believe I could live a life in control of my problems.
>
> (Lovejoy, 1984: 812)

> I want to feel heard and understood. I want to know about my options, and I want to be supported to make a decision based on what matters to me.
>
> (Anonymous service user, NHS England, 2013: 13)

> I needed a safe place – somewhere I could not seriously harm myself until I recovered emotionally. I also needed to feel that someone actually cared about me . . .
>
> (Anonymous service user, Mind, 2011: 2)

Often traditional approaches have relied upon care being prescribed by experts (see Chapter 1). This undermines a collaborative and interactive approach, where the service user is involved as an active participant. Power differences in relationships can lead to submissive concordance, or passive resistance from service users. Often it is remarked that service users take little interest in participating in their care plan, and so this process is completed for them, which leads to a loss of autonomy and feelings of disempowerment on the part of the service user. In many ways this is the antithesis of recovery, as the whole process robs the service user of the capacity for self-determination and making choices in life. Often in mental health settings, especially inpatient wards, the staff lose interest in promoting recovery because it is felt that the service users lack interest and enthusiasm. Perhaps their experience of the system leads them to feel bereft of motivation through not being involved in care, or made to feel that it is outside of their influence. To arrive at truly collaborative solutions, there needs to be an emphasis on promoting empowerment, actively engaging the service user and jointly exploring problems. This has more meaning and therapeutic value for the person, and so it is likely that they will feel more motivated to participate in their care.

Understanding how the person experiences the problem is essential in a recovery-influenced approach. Yet for this to be genuine, professionals need to accept that the service user has to have the right to be able to select the choices that we might not prefer. Often this is the sticking point between accepting recovery and carrying it out in practice, as there is the temptation to take back control when the service user prefers the choice we would not wish them to make. Understandably this leaves service users feeling not listened to, or that the philosophy of recovery is not evident in practice.

Exercise

Q: Have you experienced a situation in life when you did not feel listened to?

How did this make you feel?

Ensuring that the service user's perspective is listened to is essential, even if there are not ready-made solutions.

Now think of a situation when you felt listened to.

Contrast this with the above experience. What were the differences in how the interaction felt for you? What made the difference in feeling listened to or not?

A: In any relationship, personal or professional, effective communication is essential if the relationship is to be healthy and productive. There are various ways in which we can tell whether we are 'being heard'. For example, we know if someone is listening to us by their verbal responses, but also through more subtle signs, including body language, eye contact and tone of voice (see Chapter 3).

Now consider what you can take forward and emulate in your own practice working with service users.

Being listened to, having the time to express needs, and receiving affirmation, validation and reassurance are vital elements in a supportive care relationship. It is hoped that interactions with mental health nurses support and facilitate service users in gaining and cultivating a sense of hope and choice, within a safe and supportive environment to assist their path to recovery. The concept of hope plays a vital role in mental and physical well-being. Without hope the need for a person to want a future is very limited:

> Hope is what makes us human, if I wasn't given hope for the future – what future would I have had?
>
> (Anonymous service user, 2015)

To help and support the service user to build hope, it is paramount to provide stability, support and time. Listening is a skill (see Chapter 3 on communication) and active listening on the part of the mental health nurse allows the service user to express their thoughts in a manner that can help to identify and work through problems but also recognize and gain confidence in strengths and skills. It may seem easy to understand what it means to care for a person, but providing skilled care requires patience, perseverance and a commitment to the service user. Often the competing demands of the professional role of the mental health nurse can lead to paperwork, documentation and bureaucracy taking precedence over time spent with the service user. It is often remarked upon by students that the work of mental health nurses involves a disappointing emphasis on paperwork (see Chapter 5). Although these aspects of a person's care are also essential, they should be secondary to the core purpose of supporting the person in crisis.

Example 1

Imagine you are a male, who has just been diagnosed with schizophrenia at the age of 28. You are unsure what this diagnosis means and how people are going to react to this life-changing issue. Your wife and family know that you have sought help but how do you tell them? You are likely to have many questions about your future, for example, what is going to happen with your career? Potential feelings you may experience are: anxiety, fear, confusion and frustration. At this point, consider whether you would feel able to attend to your basic needs such as eating, drinking and caring for your personal hygiene. Are you likely to feel sociable and be able to carry on with your normal daily routine? These are all aspects of a person's life that can be affected by a mental health diagnosis. One service user describes their experience of being diagnosed with schizophrenia:

> It felt like the end of the world when I was diagnosed with schizophrenia 20 years ago. Before that, I had a really full life – I worked hard, had lots of friends, and was always out partying. But according to the psychiatrist, all that seemed to be over. I was told that I'd never be able to have children or work again, and I thought to myself, 'I don't want this schizophrenia!'. . .
>
> (Service user, Rethink, 2013: 6)

Example 2

For your entire life you have felt 'different from others', regularly experiencing intense and unpredictable emotions throughout your adolescent years and into adulthood. At the age of 24 you receive a diagnosis of BPD (see explanation of BPD below). You have no idea what this is, though the term suggests that there is something wrong with your personality. You start to feel hopeless and you begin to remember various encounters where you felt that people have judged you negatively. The emotions are overwhelming and you cannot make sense of them. You may swing rapidly between feelings: you may be lethargic and have little energy and interest in doing anything, or you may feel angry and distressed. This, in turn, may affect your ability to attend to your basic needs and potentially stop you from wanting to undertake activities that you would normally enjoy. For some people, knowing they have a mental health problem can be reassuring and explains why they may have experienced problems that other people do not. The person may benefit from the support of family, friends and the mental health services. However, it may still take time and there can be significant and traumatic consequences as a result of this possibly life-changing event.

Working all of the time with people who are diagnosed with severe and enduring mental health problems can lead mental health nurses to become desensitized to the needs of service users when coming to terms with a diagnosis. To help us work more effectively and empathically, it is worth reflecting on the significant adjustment the person undergoes. The impact of being diagnosed with a mental health problem is described in this next comment from a service user.

> I just found myself waking up and not being able to get out of bed anymore. I was so tidy and house-proud before I got depression and I just no longer cared about anything. I lost my job – probably because I didn't tell them what was going on and just kept getting warnings for not turning up. I just lost myself and any hope in life. My family didn't understand, they just said things like 'pull yourself together' – like I hadn't already thought of that.
>
> (Anonymous service user, 2016)

It is important when a person has just been diagnosed with a mental health problem that they are given information on the condition. It also helps for the person to talk and to express their issues: fears, expectations and perceptions. Providing positive but realistic views of how life can still continue successfully, even with a major mental health problem, may come as a reassurance. When offering health information, it is tempting to comprehensively equip the person with everything that it is possible to know. However, it is necessary to consider whether the person is able to comprehend, or even wants large amounts of information that may or may not be useful and relevant.

If I have just been told that I have a mental health problem that is probably the biggest and most significant news that I need to know. There may be some other things I would like to know, or that is a legal, or Trust requirement but as the mental health nurse acting to support the person, it is worth considering the context of the situation, what the person says they want. It is also important to answer questions specifically, rather than giving lengthy or falsely optimistic information to appease the person. Answering questions truthfully, honestly and realistically though also tactfully and sensitively will help. Through this conversation we may also understand whether the service user has preconceived ideas about what they expect people with mental health issues to be like. Also whether they have certain beliefs about healthcare, for example, whether there are effective evidence-based treatments. Furthermore, we may come to know what treatment options they might prefer.

We need to avoid jargon, technical terms and 'buzzwords'. If the service user is in agreement, it can be helpful to actively involve families, carers and significant others in care (see example in Chapter 5). Families, carers and significant others often provide an indispensable resource in supporting the service user, and as mental health nurses, we have an obligation to assess and provide a plan of care for those close to the service user. Often families and carers have fears and anxieties that may be alleviated with information, education, support and even inclusion in the care process (see Chapter 8).

Exercise

Consider when you have been given significant news relating to health. It may have been delivered to you personally, or you may have been present and involved with a family member or significant other. The healthcare professional can be from any discipline or level of seniority.

Consider what made the communication good or bad.

What else might the person have done, or what did they do to make you feel supported?

Do you feel that the person's profession was influential in how they provided support for you?

What can you take from reflecting on this example, in terms of it inspiring you and being practice that you wish to emulate, or that you want to do better for your service user? Write this down in your portfolio as a personal goal.

In the next part of the chapter, we look at stigma, specifically in relation to a service user with BPD.

Stigma within mental health services

Service users are often well aware of being treated differently by staff because of their mental health issue. Over a number of years, researchers have considered whether certain service users are viewed more negatively due to their diagnosis (Link et al., 1987). As far back as the 1960s, it was recognized that mental health practitioners had negative perceptions towards certain mental health conditions (Link et al., 1987; Markham, 2003). Some service users find mental health services to be indifferent to their needs and experiences.

> Yeah the attitudes can be quite difficult because they can't place you, it's not like I'm a schizophrenic or you've got this very definite problem . . . I think that they think that you're being difficult most of the time, I know they think 'Oh God, she's playing up'.
>
> (Anonymous service user, Fallon, 2003: 397)

It could be argued that it is the case that there is an overreliance on 'labelling' and diagnosis, which, in turn, can create an expectation of certain behaviours. This can lead to the person only being seen in terms of their mental health problem:

> I feel that when I tell staff my diagnosis they look at me differently, probably just thinking that I'm mad and they don't take my feelings seriously.
>
> (Anonymous service user, 2016)

> Because I have a mental health diagnosis, everyone thinks that when I get upset or say something isn't right, it must be because I'm becoming 'unwell' again and not that I'm actually reacting in a normal way to something . . . I get scared they'll put my medication up.
>
> (Anonymous service user, 2016)

Many people with a diagnosis of BPD report especially negative experiences with staff (Bonnington and Rose, 2014; Horn et al., 2007). It has been suggested that service users are well aware of these prejudices that often lead to an increase in challenging behaviours and, in turn, further reinforcing stigma and negative attitudes on the part of staff (Link et al., 1987; Markham, 2003). Within the Mental Health Act of 1983 BPD was not classified as a diagnosis (Legislation. gov.uk., 1983; Thomson, 2010). Although the reform of the Mental Health Act in 2007 did identify BPD as a distinct and treatable diagnosis (Legislation. gov.uk, 2007), many practitioners still dispute such symptoms even being classified as a mental health problem (Sen and Irons, 2010; Tyrer, 2009; Wahl and Aroesty-Cohen, 2010).

BPD is a cluster of behaviours typified by an unstable sense of self, emotions and relationships with other people (*Diagnostic and Statistical Manual of Mental Disorders* (DSM-5) (American Psychiatric Association, APA, 2012). Sometimes it is referred to as *emotionally unstable personality disorder*. BPD refers to the distinction between neurosis and psychosis.

Guidelines classify people with BPD to have problems with:

- intense and unstable interpersonal relationships;
- disturbed perceptions of self-identity;
- unpredictable fluctuations in mood;
- episodes of extreme hopelessness and despair;

- acute fear of abandonment and rejection;
- reckless, impulsive and seemingly detrimental behaviour;
- illogical surges of anger, or difficulties regulating anger;
- expressed intent, threats or acts of self-harm;
- transitory symptoms of psychosis, including: paranoia, delusions, hallucinations and disassociation.

> (Bateman and Krawitz, 2013; National Institute for Health and Care
> Excellence (NICE), 2009; Norman and Ryrie, 2013;
> World Health Organization (WHO), 2010)

BPD is believed to be caused by a variety of biopsychosocial factors (Bateman and Krawitz, 2013; Mind, 2015). Problems in childhood, including abuse, are thought to play a part, with those diagnosed with BPD often having a history of key developmental experiences including:

- trauma;
- physical, sexual or emotional abuse;
- chronic fear or distress;
- abandonment;
- neglect;
- enduring feelings of instability during developmental milestones;
- a higher degree of mental health disorders within the family genogram.

> (Bateman and Krawitz, 2013; Grosjean and Tsai, 2007;
> Mind, 2012; NICE, 2009; Wrycraft, 2012)

BPD is characterized by the '3Ps': it is persistent, problematic and pervasive. **Persistent** refers to continuing and repeated problems. For example, a service user has a string of abusive relationships, all with similar features. The diagnosis is **Problematic** in terms of causing major inconvenience and distress; and finally it is **Pervasive** in being apparent in different areas of the person's life. People with BPD often have chaotic personal relationships, financial affairs, and work/education difficulties.

Unsurprisingly, people with BPD also often experience other mental health issues. These include:

- anxiety;
- eating disorders;
- depressive disorders;
- post-traumatic stress disorder;
- bipolar disorder;
- substance misuse.

> (Bateman and Krawitz, 2013; Mind, 2012;
> NICE, 2009; Wrycraft, 2012)

In spite of these highly significant factors, some people with BPD recover in time (NICE, 2009). Studies have shown 85 per cent of individuals with BPD will not meet the diagnostic criterion 10 years after diagnosis (Mind, 2015). It has been suggested that this may not always be down to treatment, but that change occurs over time that enables the learning of effective psychological skills (Bateman and Krawitz, 2013; Zanarini, 2008).

Exercise

Q: Is BPD is a discrete mental health issue in its own right? Or is it a disparate collection of symptoms and features, grouped together for the convenience of healthcare staff to be able to label and diagnose service users?

A: On the one hand, diagnosis allows us to create treatment pathways and therapeutic interventions for this group of service users. On the other hand, the wide range of challenging behaviours within this diagnosis means that it is almost inevitable that these service users will become an unpopular group among those who care for them. It is not surprising that service users who are diagnosed with BPD experience stigma and discrimination and are unpopular within the mental health services.

Research suggests mental health nurses have limited knowledge of BPD. It is suggested that mental health nurses do not understand how service users feel about their diagnosis, how they cope with their stressors, or what their experiences are with the mental health services (Bonnington and Rose, 2014; Sheenan et al., 2016). This lack of knowledge seems to be a key factor contributing to the development of stigma (Bonnington and Rose, 2014; Sheenan et al., 2016). Mental health nurses can also lack the specialist skills required to address the often challenging needs of service users with BPD. The behaviours of people with BPD can adversely affect those around them, for example, they may develop very close relationships with some members of staff, but reject others, which can lead to 'splitting' and attempts at manipulation within ward teams. Often these issues expose resource and training limitations that are expressed in terms of resentment of people with BPD.

Q: Looking at the above, and reflecting on your own practice experience, how might we improve this situation?

A: Negative attitudes can be challenged through effective clinical supervision. This process provides support to mental health teams, to enable them to cope effectively and compassionately with the challenging and complex needs and behaviours of people with BPD. The development of specialist resources to provide appropriate treatment and care for this group of service users is also helpful. In addition to this, providing specialist training to mental health nurses in therapeutic approaches, such as dialectical behavioural therapy (DBT), which research shows to be an effective treatment for BPD, will help them feel better equipped to work with people with these issues. Education on what the diagnosis of BPD means for people, and the experiences encountered on a daily basis, can help in developing empathy and understanding on the part of mental health nurses (Bonnington and Rose, 2014; Fallon, 2003; Horn et al., 2007).

In light of this, there are two case studies below which explore the experiences that people with BPD have encountered within the mental health services (see Table 6.1 at the end of the case studies).

Case Study 6.1   BPD: community service experience

Amy is a 19-year-old girl who is currently feeling hopeless in her life. Amy has a diagnosis of BPD and has been in contact with community mental health services intermittently over the past five years. She feels as though her Community Mental Health Nurse (CMHN) is not taking her feelings and experiences seriously and is starting to feel like no one cares. She is questioning whether there is any point in living a life feeling this way.

Amy has a lot of overwhelming feelings that she struggles with on a daily basis:

> I get intrusive thoughts that just take me over. They're criticizing thoughts: asking me why I am bothering with my life because no one cares, no one loves me, I'm stupid, I won't get anywhere in my life. No one understands.

Amy described having a difficult childhood, growing up around verbally and physically abusive parents, though she will not elaborate on these experiences. She describes herself as being the 'ugly sister' and bullied throughout her school life due to the way she looked. She found learning at school very hard and felt that her teachers and family thought she was 'just stupid' and didn't care about her education, rather than helping her.

> I hated school, the bullies, the work, the teachers; I found it really hard to learn and I felt like no one cared – I started to believe I was stupid but also felt that there was something else wrong with me. I wanted to learn, I found a lot of things very interesting but I just couldn't understand things.

At the age of 13 Amy started having various unstable, intense and destructive relationships. She said that one of her relationships ended because of physical and emotional abuse, as well as infidelity by her boyfriend. At this time she started to drink a lot of alcohol after school and at the weekends and became promiscuous with older men.

> Drinking for a few hours made me feel better about myself and stopped me caring what others thought of me. I wanted boys to like me – it made me feel better about myself.

Amy states that during relationships she always finds herself comparing her looks to other girls of her age:

> I find me comparing myself to others. Everyone looks better than me. Why can't I look like them? Why would anyone want to be with me?

At the age of 13 Amy also began to self-harm: cutting her arms, wrists, inner thighs; biting her nails and inner mouth. She also would not eat except when her parents forced her but after the meal induced vomiting, which resulted in a significant weight loss. At the age of 14 Amy wanted to end her life and took an overdose.

> I had had enough of this world; I wrote a letter to my family – took the pills and went to sleep hoping that I wouldn't wake up.

This is when Amy first came into contact with the mental health services and was referred by her GP to a counsellor. Amy said that she really liked her counsellor:

> She was the first lady I felt really cared for me and I looked forward to seeing her every week. I was really sad that after having a certain amount of sessions I wasn't allowed to see her anymore because otherwise I'd get too attached to her – I don't know why – and then I was just left alone again.

At the age of 18, Amy was seen by a psychiatrist every 3–6 months and was put on medication to assist in stabilizing her mood. During this time, she was also referred to a Community Mental Health Team where she first met her CPN.

> I think she feels that I'm just being pathetic when I cry. She kind of has the attitude of 'oh, here she goes again'. She clearly doesn't like me. I just started to feel more stupid and just proved my point that no one cares about me.

> All I want is for someone to listen to me and to actually listen to what I'm saying. Do people think I want to feel like this? Do people think that I want to be like this?

> I want to get on with my life and make something of myself. Why don't people take me seriously? It's hopeless.

Q: How have staff attitudes affected Amy?

A. It is evident that Amy feels as though her CMHN does not care about her and what she is experiencing. These feelings have triggered emotional turmoil that has now escalated her beliefs into thoughts that 'no one' cares for her.

Q: What does Amy need?

A: Amy wants to be listened to and cared for. Amy appears to have lacked stability in her life, especially during her childhood during her development. As a result, she lacks trust and hope in people that she should be able to rely on and is continually afraid of abandonment and/or rejection.

Q: How could Amy's care have been handled differently?

A: Amy feels that her CMHN has been invalidating her experiences. This has exacerbated Amy's sense of hopelessness for her future. When Amy is relating her experiences, it is essential for her CMHN to validate, reassure and actively listen to her. This will provide Amy with the consistency and stability that she has lacked in her life, which has resulted in her continuous fear of dismissal. NICE (2009) guidelines suggest people with BPD such as Amy require structure and continuity in their care. This would allow Amy to work with her CMHN to build confidence and develop adaptive coping mechanisms to enable her to manage challenging situations.

Case Study 6.2   BPD: inpatient service experience

Jake is a 27-year-old man who is experiencing a crisis. Jake lacerated his neck after taking a large amount of heroin. His neighbours heard loud music in the early hours of the morning and called the police who found Jake in his bedroom, semi-conscious and bleeding profusely. Jake was taken to A&E and when physically stable was assessed by the crisis team and admitted informally to an inpatient mental health unit. Jake agreed to the admission as:

> If I go home I don't know what will happen, I don't feel safe. I don't want to hurt myself but I don't see any way out.

Jake describes a 'living nightmare' childhood. He said that he was taken into care around the age of six due to his mother not being mentally well enough to care for him.

> She was drinking a lot and crying all the time. I don't really remember too much or want to. I just remember growing up feeling alone. I never knew my Dad. I was given foster parents but they didn't care. Then I got into drugs and alcohol with the wrong sort of people, I guess you'd say. Drugs and alcohol make me feel better though; it's like an escape that you want more and more.

Jake reported first taking drugs at the age of 15 and now appears to be a dependent user. Jake reported that all of his friends are drug users and this is how he has met all of his girlfriends. He has described having intense and unstable relationships, often ending in violence from both sides. He describes struggling with his emotions and often getting irritable and angry over things and feeling unable to control his emotions.

> Me and Zoe (his girlfriend) often have bad arguments, I don't even know why. She just really winds me up sometimes and then I hit the wardrobes or the wall which then upsets her more. What am I meant to do? I'm in a lose-lose situation with her.

Jake describes often getting thoughts about killing himself and then takes drugs to help 'block the thoughts out'. Jake states that he does not work and lives in a council-owned flat.

> I've never worked; I didn't do well at school so no one would want me work-ing for them – I'm useless. I was always suspended from school, none of the teachers cared and my foster parents just had a go at me all the time. I moved into my friend's house, sleeping on his sofa at 18 and it just went from there.

Jake stated that he has been having more extreme thoughts of ending his life for the past six months (since becoming 27) and while Zoe was away at a festival, he thought he would use this opportunity to act on these thoughts.

> I felt like I wanted to die but I'm not sure now, I just felt everything was so pointless and I always mess everything up. I was surprised that anyone cared enough to save me – but I guess it's just their (the policeman's) job.

When Jake was admitted onto the ward, he was seen by the consultant who gave him a diagnosis of BPD.

> I think knowing what's wrong with me has helped, I don't feel so clueless in why I'm like this now but I would like to know more about it. But I've heard quite a few patients on the ward saying that the nurses don't like people like me.

> Since being here I can tell that most of the nurses don't like me and the other patients were right. I think they think that I'm a waste of time. I can just tell by their attitudes, you know? But there is one nurse, she's meant to be my main nurse. She listens to me and seems to actually care – makes a change! But I'm sure she's only doing it because she has to . . . Still at least someone cares enough to pretend they like me. I think the rest of them just think that I'm doing it for attention or something – but this nurse is different, she's making me feel better about myself and she's giving me lots of stuff to read about positive thinking. We've even been discussing what jobs I could do when I get out of here.

Q: How have staff attitudes affected Jake?

A: Jake's story highlights the impact of how mental health nurses can support a person's well-being and how compassionate care can support people's hope in their future. Jake stated that he encountered nurses who gave him the impression that they did not care, which was corroborated by fellow service users. While saying this, he also clearly identified his keyworker (main nurse) as someone who is supporting his needs; listening to him and is promoting positivity concerning his future.

Q: What does Jake need?

A: Similar to Amy's story, Jake wants to feel wanted and listened to. He lacked stability in his early years, which may have contributed to him developing unhealthy relationships in adulthood. At crucial points in his childhood Jake lacked stable parent figures to act as positive role models and has not developed self-esteem and feels like he is 'useless' in life.

Q: How could Jake's care have been handled differently?

A: Upon admission to the inpatient ward, Jake was made to feel unwelcome by mental health nurses who have given him the impression that they do not care about what he is currently experiencing. In contrast with Amy's story, though, Jake has a positive relationship with his keyworker.

Exercise

From what you have read in this chapter and your practice experience, how do you feel about people with BPD now?

If your perceptions are negative, how might they become more positive? Think about skills you might learn, or approaches to practice that might produce different or more constructive responses from service users.

Due to the nature of their problems, people with BPD may present significant challenges for mental health services. Mental health nurses often feel that they lack the necessary skills, training and support to deal with some of the issues. As a result service users with BPD may be avoided or ignored and receive less effective care from mental health nurses than other groups of service users. Mental health nurses may be better equipped to deal with these challenges by regular staff and multidisciplinary team (MDT) support that allows the input of other professionals such as psychologists. This allows teams to deal with issues collectively and collaboratively. Regular training and updates on BPD and post-registration training in specific therapeutic approaches in

Table 6.1 Shared factors that both Amy and Jake needed from their care

Validation	Respect
Care	Empathy
Stability	Safety
Consistency	Compassion

working with people with this mental health problem will better equip staff in meeting these challenges.

Conclusion

In this chapter we have considered the perspective and needs of service users. In many of the quotes that have been presented, and in the case studies, service users' own words have been used, to better represent their lived experiences. In practice, wherever possible, it helps to enter into the language of service users and avoid technical jargon and terminology. This not only prioritizes and empowers the service user but reminds us we are dealing with real people and very real issues.

Within the chapter there has been a particular emphasis on BPD, as it is sometimes suggested that this is a source of discrimination and unpopularity among mental health nurses. Often we talk about stigma and discrimination in the past tense: while the situation has certainly improved, there is still evidence of deeply entrenched negative attitudes towards people with this diagnosis. If we are to develop as people and practitioners, we must continually reflect and openly and honestly challenge our own attitudes and beliefs. Understanding service users' views helps mental health nurses develop empathy and a less defensive view towards what are undeniably very often difficult issues.

7 Recovery and multidisciplinary working

Nick Wrycraft

In any area of mental health services, we will be working in the delivery of care together with other professionals and agencies. As a result of the deinstitutionalization of mental health services over the last 30 years, but also the focus of government policy for health generally, there is now an emphasis on delivering services in the community (NHS England, 2017). In the future this will be a more important feature of our work more than ever.

Over the years there have been numerous cases from Victoria Climbie to Baby P where multiple agencies have failed to work together to share information that would permit the early detection of problems (HM Government, 2003; Local Safeguarding Children Board (LSCB) Haringey, 2009). These are the headline-grabbing cases and deservedly so, but there are innumerable less prominent though no less unacceptable instances of poor communication or co-ordination of services that lead to service users losing out, or their needs being overlooked or neglected. As the professionals most directly involved in the delivery of mental healthcare to service users, nurses need to work effectively alongside and in collaboration with other services in co-ordinating care. Developing skills in managing and using these relationships to their optimal potential is an essential skill set for student mental health nurses to acquire.

For the most part multidisciplinary teams (MDTs) perform a positive and useful role in moving the care of service users forward with the input of all parties. Sometimes though there can be challenges. There may be rivalries between different professional disciplines, or teams, especially where services are stretched, under-resourced and feel burdened. Or there may be differences in perception of what the input of the MDT ought to be in a specific service user's care. In some other cases aspects of the relationship between the service user and services may be mirrored in the relationships between the members of the MDT, and a parallel process occurs (Hawkins and Shohet, 2012). For example, a service user who is very reluctant to engage with services and who is hostile may have an MDT where there are arguments and fractures in the relationships between the professionals involved in their care. Alternatively, a service user who is highly anxious and afraid of any kind of threat or risk may have an MDT that is peculiarly risk-averse.

The mental health nurse's role in working in the MDT is flexible and adaptable. We may be a diplomat acting as the go-between for professionals who do not agree on the right course of action, or who are advocating different solutions. Or we may be a negotiator brokering a deal between services who view the same situation from a completely different perspective due to their differing culture and outlook. At other times we may be a leader and pulling together disparate services who all input into the service user's care, but no one seems able or willing to take control. We may also be a counsellor and supporting an exasperated MDT who are bereft of ideas to help a service user who has exhausted all of the available options. Working to make the MDT function will ensure that care is effective and responsive and that there is fluid and co-ordinated communication and shared decision making. It is helpful to reflect upon the dynamics of these relationships in terms of:

- What has contributed to creating the current working relationship?
- What crucial action(s) do we need to take to move things forward?
- What is the desired outcome?

Often progress is stifled by resistance, people being stubborn or specific health-care providers not sharing a common goal which always ought to be to move the service user's care forward and promote recovery. In this chapter we consider some of the specific skills that mental health nurses use with regard to MDT working and recovery-focused practice. Readers will consider:

- What is the MDT, and how can we use it to practise in a recovery-focused manner?
- How can mental health nurses promote MDT working?
- How can we improve how we used MDT working in developing practice?

MDT

MDT working is where a group of health, allied health and medical profession-als consider different treatments and work together collaboratively to develop and implement care plans for service users (Ke et al., 2013). Sometimes mental health nurses or other health professionals, for example, a physiotherapist, may both have input into the same service user's care, yet due to the nature of their work there may be no need for mutual co-operation or collaboration. MDTs are established where the input of different agencies, professionals or specialisms overlap. Another advantage of the MDT, however, is to work out-side the boundaries and confines imposed by the normal ways of working, through accessing the specialist knowledge, skills and best practice from numerous services working in different disciplines (NHS England, 2014).

MDT working commonly occurs in adult nursing in the care of older people, critical care heart disease and stroke, but are also highly prevalent throughout mental healthcare (Ke et al., 2013). This may be because of the nature of mental healthcare, meaning that the input of different healthcare professionals overlap. Also that users of acute mental health service users are often involved with other healthcare agencies and professionals. People with physical health issues are more prone to experience mental health issues, while mortality rates due to acute physical health issues are higher among people with mental health issues (British Medical Association (BMA), 2014; Mental Health Foundation (MHF), 2011, Royal College of Psychiatrists (RCP), 2010).

Many mental health nurses value working closely alongside other professionals from different disciplines. This form of interpersonal, mutually respectful, sharing of knowledge, experience and collaborative working demonstrates a high level of professionalism and carrying out what we have trained to do in action. Often the discussions that occur are robust and vigorous. Yet the focus is always on benefiting the service user's recovery, and choosing the best option rather than winning the argument. It is this that makes MDT working in mental healthcare so highly fulfilling and rewarding, and where carried out successfully is an essential contributing factor to promoting recovery for service users.

Q: Reflect back on your practice placement experience. What might be some of the problems with different disciplines involved in the care of one service user?

A:
- Some professionals might not be aware of the involvement of others.
- There might be overlap. For example, a mental health nurse and social worker might both be helping the service user with their finances, yet unaware of each other's involvement. The service user may assume that the professionals are already communicating.
- Due to their differing professional perspectives, the involvement of multiple professionals has the potential to produce contradictory or different approaches. For example, in the case of an older person with limited mobility and who has returned home after a hip replacement. The mental health nurse might encourage them to mobilize just enough in order to complete everyday tasks without overextending their capability and exposing themselves to risk. In contrast, the physiotherapist may encourage the service user to mobilize much more, and to stretch their capabilities in order to rehabilitate completely. The contrast between approaches may be to the extent that one profession actively disapproves of, or feels the other approach to be risky, irresponsible, or overlooking other important information.
- The profession taking the lead in determining care may not be the service that has the most input into care, understanding of the case, or relevance

to the service user's need(s). Often the medical profession take charge and responsibility for driving the MDT. Yet if this is a case where medication is less significant, or other professionals have important contributions to make, it may be better that they lead the discussion. Consequently, all of the professions involved ought to receive equal input, or at least an opportunity to influence decisions, so that all of the relevant information and viewpoints are shared, and a truly collaborative approach can be taken.

- The service user may relate differently to some professionals than others. It is often the case that there can be widely different impressions between professionals of the level of dependence or independence of the service user. This may be because some assessments reveal a greater level of need than others. However, the service user may respond differently to different individuals or approaches, leading to differing impressions being formed. In some cases professionals from the same discipline may form a different impression of the service user's level of need. Yet rather than being seen as problems these issues ought perhaps to be seen as opportunities for the MDT to engage and discuss these differences, and seek explanations as to why this is the case.

Q: Looking at the aspects above, what can we learn in terms of the factors that make good MDTs?

A:
- Open and inclusive sharing of information.
- Combining expertise and utilizing the professional skills and training of the team.
- Equality and the active promotion of shared ownership of the MDT.
- Power or professional hierarchy not being used to give one group's views greater prominence.
- Shared responsibility for decisions between the professionals.
- Sharing the workload evenly between the contributing members of the MDT.
- Active and collaborative involvement of the service user at all points.
- Seeking feedback from the service user.
- Inviting contrasting perspectives and options for therapeutic interventions and strategies.
- An approach that emphasizes continuous learning, and the sharing of up-to-date practice.
- Adaptability and involving services flexibly around the needs of the service user.
- Wanting to continuously improve.
- Members of the team supporting one another.

Exercise

Look at the above factors. In your practice experience on placement, have you seen some or all of these at work?

Did they enhance the service user's care?

Communication between different professionals is the oxygen that allows the MDT to carry out its everyday role. In the event of emergencies, and where the person is experiencing crisis, this becomes especially important in responding rapidly and effectively to changing circumstances. In order for this to be achieved, there needs to be good working relationships and established routes and patterns of communication.

Good communication ensures that:

- Care can be planned and strategized. For example, where multiple professions have input into the service user's care, it can be agreed when and at what intervals individual services will be involved and what the expected outcome will be.
- Where communication is good, it is easier to identify problems if things go wrong and care is seamless. Overall, the service user will feel that they are involved with one service rather than several. Their care can be more personalized and individual than if they are dealing with different professionals from different organizations.
- Often different services have their own systems, ways of working and bureaucracy that can cause confusion. The MDT working together and sharing information overcomes bureaucracy and acts to minimize the inconvenience of, for example, problems and delays with service users being referred between services.
- Trained professionals from different disciplines can work with and alongside each other to share professional expertise, experience and approaches to practice in agreement with the service user.
- Mutual support is available between professionals, which is useful in offsetting stress and any problems in the relationship with the service user's care.
- Shared responsibility between trained professionals may ensure that there is less potential for blame when things go wrong.
- Good communication within the MDT may avoid individual professionals being excessively burdened or taking too much responsibility or having more input in the service user's care than is reasonable.

Case Study 7.1   Nora

Nora is 78 years old and experiencing chronic obstructive pulmonary disease (COPD). She lives with her husband Stan. Nora is also entering the terminal stages of cancer but refusing to go into a hospice for care. She receives a comprehensive package of care including the community-based COPD team and Macmillan nurses. Recently Nora took an accidental overdose of medication, because she is on numerous tablets and could not keep track of what she had and had not taken.

When reading the case notes in Nora's home, a member of the COPD team on a routine visit realizes that the mental health team are also involved because Nora has become depressed and has been prescribed anti-depressant medication. In a group clinical supervision session meeting (see Chapter 5), the team discussed various aspects of this issue, and were concerned at the lack of co-ordination of the multiple services involved in Nora's care without mutual consultation. It was also felt that the team did not really understand how Nora's mental health was affecting her, and they wanted to ask the mental health service for advice. They were also concerned at how Stan was coping, as he often says he feels that he is 'at the end of his tether'. The COPD team decided to contact all of the other services involved in Nora's care to call a meeting of all of the professionals to agree a team-based approach and way forward.

This example illustrates the value of communication and necessity of working together in MDTs. It is as though everyone has some of the jigsaw but no one has the complete picture. The only way of gaining a good understanding of the whole picture, therefore, is to assemble all of the pieces together, and involve all of the services inputting care. Within mental health this may involve occupational therapists (OTs), social workers and psychologists but also, peer workers and unqualified staff, staff within the independent sector and advocates. In the wider community there may also be local government officers, such as housing and environmental health officers, and maybe police or staff in education and employment.

Working effectively within the MDT requires the ability to use and work collaboratively with other professionals and agencies to meet the service user's need(s). This calls for the use of a wide range of competences, both personal and professional. These include:

1   The ability to anticipate and respond to rapid changes in the service user's need(s). More than this, and consistent with Mary Ellen Copeland's Wellness Action Recovery Plan (WRAP) (see Chapter 11), there needs to be involvement not only with the MDT but with the service user as well. For example, where the person's mental health deteriorates and their overall functioning is impaired, it is helpful to be able to refer to a pre-existing plan that the person has agreed when well. It might be as simple as increasing the frequency of visits from the Community Mental Health Nurse (CMHN) during the period of time when the person's mood is lower; however, the process by which help or support is mobilized is important, and can be crucial in retaining the service user's willing engagement with the MDT.

2   Working innovatively and imaginatively within the team to ensure that the services meet the needs of the service user, for example, where the MDT

may routinely meet at the team's office, if the service user lives at a remote location, suggesting that the team meet there. This avoids ritualized practice. However, changes and new ideas ought to be instituted with a rationale to avoid being just change for the sake of change. Involving multiple professionals in regular team discussions about care can often provide solutions to even the most resistant and entrenched problems.

3 Often there is a loose commitment for the MDT to meet regularly, but due to pressured workloads and other priorities taking over, this does not happen. Persevering and tenaciously following through with a commitment to arrange and attend regular meetings are essential. The Care Programme Approach (CPA) is a necessary and binding commitment on the mental health services, and exists as a result of historical shortfalls in services to both support people with mental health issues and safeguard the public. So while the CPA is often seen as placing a bureaucratic burden upon services, it exists for a very good reason, and the opportunity to engage with other agencies and professionals provides the opportunity to foster closer team-working and co-operation. Anecdotally, in practice, there is often a perception that it is a waste of time sending invitations to MDT meetings or CPA reviews to certain professionals because they do not attend. Care is enhanced, however, by the active participation and sharing of communication between all parties, and so even where the professional to whom you are writing is unlikely to attend, it is still good practice to invite them.

4 Mental health nurses bringing agencies together in the care of service users, either through making referrals or simultaneously being involved in care together with other professionals. It is necessary that we take time to reflect on our experiences when engaging with other professionals, so that our communication can develop and is congruent with those with whom we engage, professional and demonstrates values and principles consistent with recovery. Often different agencies and organizations have specific rules and cultures, and it can be disconcerting and even disempowering to open dialogue with other professionals where the cultural norms are very different from those we have learned. Part of becoming a qualified practitioner is understanding and appreciating these issues, and through successfully negotiating these situations developing confidence and an appreciation of our skills as communicators and professionals. At times within the relationships between professionals in the MDT there may be competition, conflict or rivalry. In this situation the role of the mental health nurse is to recognize where these are occurring, and to respond professionally in a manner that overcomes divisive issues and seeks to work constructively, using practitioners' knowledge and skills in advancing the service user's care.

5 Confidence in representing the service user's viewpoint and advocating on their behalf is essential, even when dealing with more experienced professionals who may regard their view as more valid. For example, in the case of a service user who has been prescribed anti-depressant medication for the first time and after several weeks in an MDT meeting claims they are

experiencing a persistent headache since starting the medication. The doctor dismissed the notion that the headache was connected with the medication and moved on to discuss another issue. The service user seemed to be unconvinced, although did not seem to feel able to challenge the doctor. The mental health nurse who was present in the meeting noticed the service user's remaining doubt and drew the doctor's attention back to it, which resulted in continued discussion of the medication.

As we can see, working within the MDT requires confidence, intuition, knowledge, perception, skill and tact. It is likely that while on placements you will see the above displayed as they form a part of everyday interaction and are present wherever teams of people work closely together. When working as part of an MDT, a baseline of professional conduct is expected whereby individuals treat one another with courtesy, regard and respect at all times. The role of the mental health nurse is to ensure that conditions are present where members of the MDT can share their views in a supportive environment. Often behaviour that is intimidating or the misuse of power can be subtle, therefore if we feel that some professionals exert an excessive influence, or act in a manner that is disrespectful of other professions, it might be worth reflecting on what evidence leads us to this conclusion.

It is also worth remembering that effective working within the MDT does not depend on accessing as many services for the person as we can, but instead ensuring that the right ones are delivered in the right way. As with the example above, too much service involvement is confusing and disruptive for the service user, makes it difficult for them to establish positive therapeutic relationships with the different services and is also challenging to co-ordinate.

MDT meetings and the presence of multiple individuals can be intimidating for service users. It is essential, however, that service users attend or at least are consulted about the meetings and their views and preferences sought so that they can exert an influence upon their care. Preparing the service user well in advance, and discussing the upcoming meeting and the issues that need to be considered with them, ensures they have time to think and reflect upon what they want and is consistent with recovery-focused practice (Wrycraft, 2015). Planning ahead, and as with Mary Ellen Copeland's WRAP (Chapter 11), identifying the service user's preferred course of action in the event of a crisis should they not be deemed able to make a decision serves to empower the person. Where this is the case care should be taken to ensure that the service user's preferences are clearly documented. It is also important that this is communicated to the rest of the MDT, and a written and signed explanation of these preferences are available within the case-notes so that they can be easily accessed by the relevant professionals at the time they are needed. There are some limitations to this, for example, where a next of kin has power of attorney or guardianship over the service user who is not deemed to have capacity.

Central to effective MDT working is a good understanding of the roles and contribution of other professionals.

Exercise

- On practice placements spend time with other professionals and learn in detail what they do, how they carry out their role, and their specific professional perspective on practice. There may be sections of your practice document for the professional to sign and write a comment. This demonstrates breadth and depth of learning on your placement.
- Acquaint yourself with all of the available local services and agencies for service users in the community and, where possible in liaison with your mentor, contact them and arrange to make visits. Most areas have folders and a supply of leaflets available in waiting room areas. Check these are up to date, and there is a good supply of leaflets available.

Often MDT working is complex, and there can be periods of frequent contact in a short space of time with another professional or professionals over an issue relating to one particular service user. In some cases there is an expectation on one or another party to act or take responsibility. In these circumstances having a good sense of trust and a functioning and positive working relationship helps. These can be sustained through regular meetings and frequent contact, and having a clear idea about the scope and nature of each other's roles so as to be clear on mutual expectations.

Case Study 7.2   Darren

Darren is a 27-year-old-man who has been diagnosed with a schizo-affective disorder since the age of 19. The Assertive Outreach Team (AOT) has ongoing contact with Darren on a regular basis. He lives in a first floor council flat, which he feels is too small for his needs, and because of it being located upstairs and in a corner of the building makes him feel 'shut in' and 'in the dark'. Darren has applied to the council to transfer accommodation, but is regarded as being a low priority. Recently there have been complaints from his elderly neighbours about him playing loud music late at night. Unfortunately, Darren's mental health has recently deteriorated, which he feels is because of the increase in anxiety he is experiencing from living in the flat. Darren says he hears voices at night and cannot sleep, and so plays loud music to make them go away. However, due to the complaints from his neighbours the council has visited and asked him to keep the noise down, which has made Darren fearful of being evicted and this has increased his anxiety. The AOT is contacting the council housing department to discuss his situation.

Q: What issues do we need to consider in interacting with other agencies?

A: Information ought to only be shared with Darren's consent, and the discussion ought to only relate to the intended, shared purpose, which in this case concerns Darren's accommodation, as opposed to discussing more specific clinical information. Knowing the role and function of other professionals within the MDT is important, so that we have a realistic awareness and understanding of what we can expect of them and their contribution.

Case Study 7.2   Darren (*continued*)

The loud music got worse, leading Darren's neighbours to continue to complain, and the council in liaison with the AOT spoke to Darren. He said he began to feel that there was a vendetta against him and his neighbours were looking for issues to complain about him. A minor fire then occurred at the flat, following which, due to the decline in his mental state, it was felt necessary to admit Darren to an inpatient mental health unit to review his care needs, which he agreed to, and so was an informal service user. During the admission a representative from the housing department attended a ward review, and explained their concerns about the possible safety of other residents. It was eventually agreed that it might be helpful for Darren's mental health if he was moved to ground floor accommodation in a different block of flats with new neighbours. After a brief wait, a suitable flat was found. There are still occasional complaints from neighbours, and at times Darren experiences issues that cause problems but he reports feeling much happier, and has better relationships with his neighbours now.

In moving forward with Darren's care the Recovery Star has proven to be particularly useful (see Chapter 9). The Recovery Star is not specifically a multidisciplinary tool, but can be used by different mental health professionals and in collaboration with service users, as it is written in jargon-free and accessible language. The aspects it covers include a range of different functions, and it is applicable to different people with different strengths and weaknesses. For Darren, the focus of the Recovery Star on issues such as responsibilities and living skills is especially useful. The model has helped him to understand areas of his life which, if he were to take control of, might work better for him in the long term.

Exercise

Contrast how Darren's issues fit with the Recovery Star in a different way than Jodi, whose Case Study is discussed in Chapter 9.

Conclusion

MDT working offers great benefits, but also provokes specific and thought-provoking challenges. In this chapter we have considered some of the strengths and attributes required to effectively work within an MDT. Often these abilities are underestimated or taken for granted. Yet, it is necessary to apply similar skills to those used in engaging and developing therapeutic rapports with service users.

It is worth spending time learning about the roles and functions of other professionals, developing relationships, making phone calls, sending out invitations to meetings, and updating colleagues of developments in service users' care. We have also discussed the importance of advanced directives to observe the service user's wishes. All of these actions create smoothly functioning and effective networks of relationships and plans that can be used when crisis occurs.

8 Working with families, carers and significant others

Nick Wrycraft

There is no stereotypical profile for families, carers and significant others and how they engage with mental health services. I would encourage you to reflect on how we perceive and work with carers and significant others in your practice placements. Often their input is seen as an intrusion or addition to work with the service user, when it may need to be a central consideration. Often working with families, carers and significant others offers potentially huge benefits to all concerned, if only we were to use our imagination and capacity for therapeutic creativity. In this chapter we look at several examples of the experiences of partners and families. Consider how you might apply the values and principles of recovery inclusively in working with and engaging this stakeholder group. In the chapter we will consider:

- what is a carer?;
- how we might include carers in recovery-based work;
- developing our own ongoing commitment to inclusive practice through working in co-operation with carers.

The examples in this chapter have been chosen to represent a range of ages. The stage of life of a service user is extremely important, in terms of their social role and the relationships they have with others around them. Through these different stages, our needs and how we relate to others change. For example, in younger life children and teenagers are more dependent financially, socially and emotionally upon their parents or carers and the immediate family. Currently, it is common for people to have children later in life, yet also as we are all living longer, simultaneously having parents with health needs and therefore a dual caring responsibility (Pierret, 2006). As we grow up and develop, we become independent, form our own relationships and families and assume responsibilities ourselves. As we see in Chapter 9 and the Recovery Star, how we manage in relation to our responsibilities is a crucial factor in how we work towards recovery.

The effect of an individual in crisis on their extended circle of relationships is like dropping a stone in a pool of still water. Numerous ripples emanate outwards that affect the whole pool. Within mental health services, too often all that we see is the service user. We perceive the stone at the point of impact and address the crisis. The person is extracted from the situation, worked with intensively, and then returned to society and the expectation is that life resumes as normal. Yet the wider impact upon the partner, family and significant others close to the service user is frequently overlooked.

Mental health services are often reluctant to engage with families, carers or significant others. There may be a tendency to keep them at arm's length, and to just work with the service user. Perhaps this is because it is perceived that it takes extra time and energy to also work with family, carers and significant others in addition to the service user. It may also be felt that issues of confidentiality, and how much it is helpful and legal to share, make it easier to simply avoid contact with family, carers and significant others. Yet too often this is used as a convenient excuse to simply avoid engaging with these people.

The notion that in inpatient settings we work with the service user and then they are slotted back into society reflects a traditional viewpoint (see Chapter 1), which does not incorporate the influences of the community or the person's sociological setting and relationships. Mental health is more fluid and multifactorial, and in order to support service users more effectively, we need to consider relationships with family, carers and significant others and the person's wider social network. This may mean working with more people, in a wider and complex range of relationships, and relinquishing some of the power and control professionals hold. However, the potential benefits are significant. These include the possibility of sustained periods of recovery for the service user who benefits from the support of family, carers and significant others who, in turn, have had their needs considered by the mental health services.

The experience of being excluded from care can have a divisive and alienating effect on those close to the service user. They can be left with their feelings about the crisis unresolved and their relationship with the service user altered or damaged as a result of the experience. It makes the post-crisis period a fresh challenge for the service user in needing not only to process their experience of the crisis but also to resume or renew relationships with those close to them again. Or, in the worst case scenario, dealing with the loss of close relationships. Inevitably, this involves difficult feelings and emotions, which can lead to further episodes of crisis and relapse. Where carers have an ongoing commitment, there is also the danger that their needs have been neglected during the crisis and they are now expected to resume caring for the service user when they are already mentally, emotionally and physically exhausted. Many carers feel morally obliged to maintain their role and continue from a sense of duty. In the long term this can lead to resentment, and the carer losing empathy for the person they are caring for, or even resenting them as well as feeling that no one is there for them.

Q: Who might you define as a carer? How might you describe the features of people in this role?

Suggested answers: A carer is someone who provides support for another person who has a health-related need. Carers can be informal, for example, a husband, wife, partner or significant other, or a friend, neighbour or volunteer. Alternatively, the carer may be formal in the sense of working in a professional and paid capacity. They may also be a person receiving payment for a care-related service. Often we think of carers as adults, however, there are many younger carers providing support for parents (Thomas et al., 2003). Families, carers and significant others are often overlooked, or left out of the care process.

Q: Why do you think this might be the case?

Possible answers include:

- from a confidentiality point of view, the mental health services work with the service user. The Data Protection Act (1998) and the NMC Code (2015) require that information pertaining to the service user ought to be treated confidentially, or only shared with the service user's permission.
- involving family, carers and significant others may undermine the therapeutic relationship with the service user;
- some relationships have complex dynamics, and it may be difficult to involve the service user's family and wider network and be certain that this will have a positive effect. At other times, practitioners do not want to get involved for fear of the carers, family and significant others and service user turning against the mental health services, or of 'opening the floodgates' on a range of additional needs that are impossible for the scarce resources of the health services to meet.

Often for legal or other rational reasons concerning the service user's interests, it is not always possible to share information with family, carers or significant others. However, this should not drive a wedge between the services and these parties, or represent a barrier in the relationship. There are ways of engaging with family, carers or significant others that respect their viewpoint and provide support.

Exercise

Can you think of any examples from your placement experience where there has been caution in communicating with carers, family or significant others?

The role of being a carer can be mentally, emotionally and physically draining. It can be a lonely and highly responsible role that requires making difficult decisions with little certainty as to what is the right option.

Case Study 8.1 Maggie and Sam

Maggie and Sam have been together for 33 years. Sam is 77 and older than Maggie who is 72. They did not have any children, and are a quiet couple with a small but close-knit social circle. Both Sam and Maggie had good jobs working in business, and have been retired for a number of years, which they both looked forward to as an opportunity to travel and involve themselves in pursuits they had always wanted to do, such as gardening and sailing. The first sign Maggie noticed that something was not right was when Sam began to be extremely and uncharacteristically 'difficult' and argumentative over quite trivial issues, but also very suddenly prone to emotional outbursts of anger or sadness. He also very easily became tearful. Initially, Maggie put this down to boredom or a mood change that would pass but then Sam also began to be very disoriented and confused. For example, when driving the car he would forget how to operate the controls, or be uncertain where he was going. At home, Sam would put things in the wrong place and frequently lost items, when normally Sam would always know exactly where everything was. Sam also seemed to struggle with finding words and to experience increasing difficulty expressing himself. Due to the change in Sam's behaviour friends became less willing to visit and Maggie felt that 'they didn't know how to act around Sam'. Maggie persuaded Sam to make an appointment with the GP. Sam was referred for an MRI and CT scan and routine blood and urine tests and a full physical health check was carried out but no problems were found.

Maggie felt disappointed that there was no explanation found, as at least that would have identified a cause. She also described feeling guilty, believing that it was 'selfish' for her to be concerned about the loss of freedom and opportunity to engage in her leisure interests, owing to the demands of looking after Sam. Sam, on the other hand, did not feel that there was an issue and whenever Maggie tried to discuss her worries about his health, he was dismissive and flippant, saying she was worrying for no reason. Sam attended medical appointments but made it clear that this was at Maggie's insistence, and to put her mind at rest.

Sam's health and behaviour continued to deteriorate and he began to be argumentative towards other people in public places. Following a disagreement in a supermarket that Maggie described as 'highly embarrassing', she felt that she could not take Sam shopping with her anymore. Maggie was also taking on more of the domestic chores that used to be shared, and at the same time noticed Sam becoming more tired and lethargic and that he had less energy than he used to. With some persuasion and reluctance, Sam again attended the GP and further tests again provided no explanation.

Maggie felt that at some point the relationship changed from being a partnership to Sam becoming dependent upon her. Maggie believed that Sam was either unaware or in avoidance of what was happening, and so they could not have an open discussion about the issues. Maggie felt resentful because Sam still spoke as though he were able to function fully and recently had begun to plan an exotic foreign holiday that Maggie felt was totally unrealistic. Maggie felt guilty that she joined in with him planning the holiday, but secretly had no confidence they would actually make the trip.

Then Sam fell at home and broke his hip. He needed a total hip replacement, and while recuperating in the general hospital became very confused and was disruptive to the extent that he was assessed and once medically stable admitted to an elderly mental health unit. In Sam's admission information he was described as at times having been very confused, angry with ward staff, and seeming to be stressed and agitated. Maggie attended the ward review and became extremely tearful and angry. She says no one listens to her viewpoint and feels left out of Sam's care. She is frustrated that she tried so hard to draw attention to his gradual decline, but that no one listened to her until Sam was acutely unwell.

When plans for Sam to return home are discussed, Maggie says she cannot possibly cope with Sam's care, as while he has been in hospital his self-care has deteriorated. Maggie is especially upset that sometimes he needs help with feeding and on some occasions has been incontinent. Maggie says she cannot possibly care for Sam at home; however, at the same time she cannot bear to put him in full-time care as she feels this will be abandoning him and may well affect his mood.

Q: How might we respond to Maggie from a recovery-based perspective?

Suggested answers:

- Listening to Maggie's perspective supportively, so that we can understand the impact of Sam's illness upon her emotionally and how this has changed her relationship with him.
- Helping Maggie to separate out the factors that are active in her thinking so she can be aware of how she really feels. This will help her in making decisions going forward.
- Offering support and information about services that might be available to support her.
- Discussing how Maggie can respond effectively to Sam's needs.
- Reflecting back to Maggie about aspects of their relationship that still remain. For example, does he still talk about her, is he pleased to see her when she visits, and can they still enjoy one another's company?
- Invite Maggie to carers' groups on the ward, if these are appropriate.

Often working with service users engaging with family, carers and significant others is not regarded as being a necessary part of care, or is something additional that can be offered if there is time permitting. The case of Joe, on which Carole reflects in Chapter 5, represents an excellent opportunity of supporting the service user but also the family. Listening to the opinions of the family, and their experiences, and taking account of their needs are essential aspects of effective care, even if we are not able to directly help or resolve the problem. We also need to bear in mind, however, that in not all cases do carers, family and significant others have the service user's interests at heart. But supporting the service user's extended network has the potential to reinforce relationships that will promote the service user's recovery by sustaining carers in the arduous role of caring (see the example of student nurse Carole's reflection on the case of Joe in Chapter 5, p. 15). Often the input of the professionals does not need to be significant. Simply feeling listened to, recognized and acknowledged can be all that is required.

Next we look at a different example which illustrates other aspects of working with families.

Case Study 8.2 Phil

Phil is 19 years old and has been admitted to an open acute inpatient unit. He was found wandering in the town centre late at night with no shirt on or shoes and seemed to be acutely confused. He did not appear to know who he was, or where he was, and seemed to be talking to people who were not there. It was felt that Phil might have been using illicit substances. Phil's parents who he lives with report that he has been behaving strangely lately and becoming more withdrawn. Phil left school after completing his A levels, and seemed uncertain as to what he wanted to do in life. Phil's parents tried to persuade him to go to university but he was unwilling, and they felt that, together with his lack of any other alternative plan, contributed to tension in the household, and led to him becoming increasingly distant and withdrawn.

On the ward Phil was noticed to be responding to phenomena that seemed to have no basis in reality. He reported hearing voices, and sometimes attributed these to various personas, for whom he had names. He reported that conversations had occurred with them when he was on his own, or with other people. At times Phil struggled to take part in a logical conversation about a specific theme.

Phil's parents took his admission very hard and were extremely upset. They blamed themselves for putting pressure on Phil to go to university and felt these expectations had put him under too much pressure, and that this had caused his current difficulties. Phil's parents also felt angry towards his friends, believing that they had led him astray and had supplied him with illicit drugs that had contributed to the deterioration in his mental health. Phil has younger twin brothers aged 15 and has previously always enjoyed a good relationship with them but one brother has become more distant towards Phil, while the other feels that Phil always gets attention and is contributing making their parents unhappy.

As a result over time Phil's parents visited him less often on the ward and his brothers refuse to visit at all. Phil had no other visitors and often complained of feeling bored and lonely, especially when seeing other service users having visits. Phil felt let down and abandoned by his family. After some time on the ward Phil returned home for overnight leave, which did not go well as there were arguments with his brothers. His parents said that they feel anxious due to their own sense of guilt, but struggle to communicate how they feel towards him: '. . . it always comes across as we are blaming him or having a go at him – whereas we just care'. Phil says he feels unwanted at home, and that his family do not care about him or understand his mental health problem.

Phil's parents said at a multidisciplinary team (MDT) meeting that his brothers resented Phil going into hospital and felt that he had abandoned them. This mirrors Phil's feelings at their not visiting and represents a split in the family relationship. Phil's parents also said they felt a sense of loss over their son, for whom they had high hopes in terms of his life and achievements, and who they never expected would experience a mental health problem that would affect his capabilities to the extent that it has.

Q: If you were a student on placement on the ward, how might we help Phil's family using a recovery approach?

A: The ward staff might seek to develop a rapport with the family when they make contact, so that they felt able to speak openly and express their feelings. Feelings of guilt, self-reproach or shame are common for families of people with mental health issues. These take time to work through, so that they can reconcile themselves to what has happened and to prepare for the future. Talking openly and empathically with Phil's parents, if they want to have that conversation, might help them move forward in their thinking. There is no specific or set time for these feelings to last. While logically we might realize that there is no justification for the guilt, it takes time for these feelings to subside. At the moment Phil's parents find that their concern comes across as blame. We might provide encouragement to help Phil's parents communicate in a way in which Phil understands their concern, as opposed to perceiving them as blaming him.

Phil's family are supporting him as he recovers, and simultaneously having to reconcile themselves to a different perception of their son or brother. This involves developing a new relationship with Phil, and in the early stages there may be some false starts or ructions. It might be expected that leave from hospital is a positive experience. However, the experience can be complex and stressful. It can mean resuming previous roles and responsibilities, and also living up to the expectations of other people. A period of home leave not going well is not necessarily a disaster or backwards step: it might helpfully reveal an issue or concern that can be addressed. In some ways this may be positive, in the sense that those involved feel able to disclose when things are not going well. It might help for the ward staff to talk openly with the family about this, so that everyone can understand what has happened and try to see each other's viewpoint and what might be learned.

The experience of living with a person with a mental health illness is emotionally stressful and complex. We cannot simply separate the person from the problem. Instead the mental health problem is intertwined with a whole range of other factors in the life of the service user and that of their friends and family. Being a parent is a difficult responsibility, and it is often hard to know what to do to get it right. If, for example, my 14-year-old son does not want to get up in the morning for school, a range of factors may be relevant. These include:

- whether he is normally good at getting up;
- he is growing and so needs more sleep;
- he may be ill or unusually tired;
- he may be in trouble with a teacher;
- he has an exam or test that he is anxious about, or a lesson he does not like;
- he went to bed late the night before.

However, if none of the above apply and my son is normally good at getting up, I know that while I might need to be a bit firm with him, he is likely to get up with a little persuasion today and tomorrow as well. In contrast, if my son has depression and is prone to generally feeling low in the morning but has been improving recently though struggles this morning, I might experience conflicting feelings. These may include:

- desperately wanting my son to feel better and feeling upset for him;
- I may need to get to work and have other issues to attend to myself, and so feel stressed and resentful at the extra burden this additional concern places upon me;
- I may feel anxious about how best to approach the situation and unsure of what to do;
- if I leave him to sleep, and he fails to attend school, I may be in trouble with the school, and my son loses another valuable day of his education and I will blame myself if he does not pass his exams;
- I do not want to nag him, but with a bit more persuasion he might get up and feel better about himself. This might ease his depression, making it easier for him to get up tomorrow. However, he might be upset with me and this could damage our relationship.

Separating out illness-related aspects of a person's behaviour from those that are just part of their personality is impossible, and does not really help to resolve difficulties anyway. From a recovery-based perspective, the person is still the person with or without the mental health problem. They exist within the world alongside others. The philosophy of recovery suggests that we are constantly in a state of recovery and never fully well, but even when we continue to be unwell, there is always hope of improving (see Chapter 1). In the same way people, who are mentally well may behave in ways that are unusual, inconsistent or illogical. It might help for me to know that my son does not get up in the morning because he is depressed. I may then understand the immense struggle that this represents for him as opposed to him just not taking his responsibilities seriously. But it is important to recognize that the label of depression is useful for me only insofar as it helps me to understand how to approach him and that it is not just because he is lazy.

Case Study 8.3   Andy

Andy is 43 years old and lives with his wife Denise and their teenage children Emma (13) and Liam (11). Andy has had the same job for 20 years. The work is not very challenging and Andy has been able to devote considerable time and attention to his home and family. He has self-built an extension to the family home and been a 'hands-on' dad. Recently, the company was taken over and due to organizational changes Andy's whole role has changed. Andy became depressed and has been off sick from work for six weeks. During this time he has become increasingly isolated and not left the house very often. Andy has become worried that he will lose his job, not be able to pay the mortgage and the family will lose their home. In spite of reassurance from Denise, Andy could not see a way out. One day when the children were at school and Denise was at work Andy took an overdose of prescribed medication and alcohol. Denise was back later than she thought and Andy was found unconscious by the children when they came home from school. They found the tablets and alcohol beside him and called an ambulance. Denise arrived shortly afterwards.

Andy was taken to Accident and Emergency, and then following assessment was admitted to an open inpatient mental health unit. Although Andy said he wanted to end his life, and still felt that way, he agreed to remain on the ward as an informal patient and accepted treatment. Andy has been on the ward for just under a week. His mood has improved, but he still feels very low. Denise has been in every day to visit and brings personal things like clothing and books. She has been very supportive to Andy.

Q: Think about each member of the family in turn. How might they feel? When doing this, think of words to describe the emotions and feelings they are experiencing.

    Andy
    Denise
    Emma
    Liam

Suggested answers: People differ enormously in their responses. However, it helps to think about how you have formed the impression that you have. Was your response informed by

- personal experience of similar circumstances?
- seeing others react in similar circumstances in your private life?
- practice experience?

How much of your understanding was from personal experience, or an awareness of other people's experience, personally or professionally? Reflecting on this, does your perspective help or hinder you? Too much of a personal connection can lead us to feel too strongly to be helpful, while too little can lead to us not really understanding how these people feel.

Imagine you were each of the members of the family in this example, one at a time. How might they feel?

Andy
Denise
Emma
Liam

Was there any difference in your response here to the above?

If there was a difference, why might this be the case?

Here is how they felt:

Andy felt distraught at realizing what had happened. He felt immensely guilty and ashamed of his actions. He still felt low in mood during the early part of his admission. He felt helpless and powerless, in that he could not do anything to influence the outside world.

Denise felt angry with Andy for the children having seen him after his overdose. At the same time, she wondered what she had missed and regretted not having realized how unwell he must have been. She reflected on having seen his mood become progressively lower over the preceding weeks, and felt guilty at not having helped him more. She thought back to the comments he had made when he did say anything, and found a few clues in his words where he had said that life was not worth living anymore. She wished she had thought more about their meaning. As a natural optimist, Denise could not understand how Andy might feel so low. However, Denise realized Andy's mood was very low following the overdose, and kept her anger to herself when visiting him.

Emma felt a strong sense of anger towards her dad and a sense of rejection that he did not want to be alive anymore and no longer wanted to be a part of the family. She felt that her dad did not love her anymore and wondered what she had done wrong. She felt guilty that her parents had to care for her and the stress this responsibility placed them under. She also felt embarrassed. At school, she only told her best friend and no one else, and swore her to secrecy. Emma was fearful that if other people found out, they might laugh at her, and she carefully monitored her social media and the wider network to see if anything was mentioned about her dad. Dad being in hospital also meant that he could not decorate her bedroom, which upset her but also made her feel guilty for being bothered about it. When she and Liam had found dad, she had felt really scared and upset and angry with dad. He ought to be the one helping the children and not the other way round. Emma felt she just did not understand what was happening to dad.

Liam missed dad being at home. He knew dad had been sad. Dad had stopped asking him about school or football, and had not been down to the park with him for a kickabout in a long while. Liam could remember finding dad unconscious, but was not really sure why he could not wake him up. He called an ambulance as he remembered from a school assembly that when people were unconscious an ambulance ought to be called. His mum had been really pleased with him and said he had been a hero. Liam thought he was just helping his dad and wanted his family back together again.

The above accounts illustrate how the same events have deeply affected all four members of one family in different ways. Like the image of the stone in the pool with which this chapter began, one event can have ramifications for the whole family and extended network of the person. As students placed on a mental health unit, it can be hard to see the wider implications of the service user's situation. The contact we have with family members may be fleeting, but these contacts offer the important opportunity of supporting people, and of understanding the service user's situation more clearly. Brief conversations and a few supportive words can be really powerful in boosting the morale of family members, and promoting a sense of hope for them.

Sometimes mental health service users have limited family and social networks but it would be unusual for an individual to have no social relationships at all. For every service user, there will be other people who care for that person, and who are affected in some way by their difficulties. As you can see from the example of Andy, the crisis he experienced has exerted a huge effect on his family. It may take time for the family to come together and piece their relationship back together again. A process of reparation and repair needs to be undergone (see Chapter 9).

Conclusion

In this chapter we have looked at the perspective of families, carers and significant others and how mental health nurses might work productively with them in a recovery-focused manner. I suspect that some of the reluctance of services to engage with these people is through a concern that this will open the floodgates to a torrent of need that cannot possibly be met. I appreciate this concern but my underlying message is that sometimes even small acts and gestures, such as acknowledging families, carers and significant others, being receptive to their viewpoint and showing respect, contribute enormously towards helping them cope at a very challenging time.

At the same time the philosophy of recovery suggests that mental health nurses need to be aware of and prioritize returning power to the service user. It is tempting to adopt the role of mediator, broker or counsellor as with the MDT (see Chapter 7) where we can see possible potential benefits. Wherever possible, though, we need to facilitate solutions, and empower individuals by promoting supportive relationships with families, carers and significant others. Of course, this relies upon tact, discretion and judgement. Often, for example in the case of an inpatient admission, the service user may benefit from a break from the pressures of their home life. At other times it might help to encourage people to discuss issues that need to be attended to but they are avoiding. Essentially, our practice needs to be guided by discretion and the Code (NMC, 2015), working with an understanding of our own values and principles and reflecting these in our actions.

9 Taking practice forward through recovery

Nick Wrycraft

In this chapter we look at therapeutic approaches to practice that support the principles of recovery. Central to this is the notion that values and principles need to be demonstrated by our actions in practice. As we discussed in Chapter 1, if we were asked to define our values, most of us would need to stop and think about what these are, even though they are fundamental to who we are and what we do. In learning to practise in accordance with the principles of recovery we need to continually reflect, and to make conscious connections between our thoughts and actions.

The ancient Greek philosopher Socrates is said to have observed that 'A life unexamined is not worth living.' One interpretation of this comment is that life gains value and meaning through reflection. Without reflecting on our lives, both at work and personally, we cannot move forward or develop as individuals. Reflection needs to be something that we do continually. If we use reflection well, then we can better understand our own motives and how we respond in the situations that we encounter in mental health practice (see Chapter 5). However, the purpose is not only to learn so that we are better prepared when we encounter a similar situation in the future, but it is also reflection that helps us gain worth and value from our experiences. Working with people is rewarding: as mental health professionals, we are privileged to be a part of a process. Reflection allows us to fully appreciate this experience and become better at how we do it. As we become more adept and experienced as practitioners, reflection becomes a less challenging and self-conscious activity. Yet it still remains an essential element of what we do. Think ahead and imagine yourself as a mentor teaching a student mental health nurse in the future. It will be a great help to you to be able to explain in detail the rationales that underpin your actions.

In Chapters 10 and 11 we look at recovery within the structure of specific models and approaches. These include Copeland's (2015) Wellness and Recovery Action Plan (WRAP), Pearpoint's (2015) Planning Alternative Tomorrows with Hope (PATH), Barker's (2001) Tidal Model and Repper and Perkins' (2003) Psychosocial Model. These have clear and distinct features and stages. In contrast, in this chapter we adopt a more flexible approach in looking at how we can apply recovery in practice. The discussion is structured around the concept of the 3Rs of **R**isk, **R**apport and **R**eparation, which also involves restoration. The 3Rs is my own invention, and utilizes the skills derived from the values and principles we identified in earlier chapters. Alongside this, we refer to some recovery-focused tools, such as the Recovery Star and the therapeutic approach of mindfulness. Recovery is by definition a flexible and adaptable philosophy that reflects the needs of the service user and their preferences. A common theme is the development of solutions and confronting challenges, and moving forward with a new understanding.

Exercise

Please remember this exercise as you read through the rest of the chapter as we will refer to it again. Think of an activity that you were afraid of doing but that you eventually managed. Ideally, think of something from your personal life, for example, a parachute jump for charity. In most cases people feel intense fear and anxiety leading up to the event, but then afterwards a sense of relief and surprise that they ever felt so apprehensive. From the comfort of hindsight we can appreciate our own heightened sense of agitation but also satisfaction that we did not give in to our fears and decide not to go through with it.

- How did you feel beforehand?
- How did you feel afterwards?

Often service users in crisis will experience high levels of anxiety and will wonder if they have the resources to be able to meet the challenge. They may fear that they will be engulfed by their feelings. It is likely that they will be feeling stuck. The Recovery Star (MacKeith and Burns, 2011) (see below) offers a way to conceptualize this experience, and to rate it so that any change can be monitored over time. Hope is central to the concept of recovery. Often we think that having looked at all of the possibilities, a problem seems insurmountable. Coming back to it after a break or a rest may lead us to view it differently. It may even be that the mood or feeling that seemed as though it would overshadow us forever just suddenly dissipates. All that we can be certain of is that change will happen. Of course, this may improve or worsen our situation. Hopefully there will be more successes than setbacks. But there is the comfort that when we are feeling at our lowest, then something might just happen to ease the burden and make life tolerable.

Often where people find the energy to overcome one challenge, further episodes or relapses can occur and this pattern of highs and lows can feel relentless and drain our reserves of energy and hope. In this respect the experience of a mental illness is an ongoing challenge, where there may be repeated episodes and crises. My son once asked when a close relative experienced a relapse of their mental health, when will it just stop? I thought about it, and it occurred to me that part of the motivation-sapping nature of mental illness is the relentlessness with which it recurs. All that we can do in the face of this potentially engulfing force is to cling on. Episodes of relapse might be seen as individual battles in an overall war.

I have used the notion of reparation as an aspect of recovery, because it demonstrates hope being thrown like a beacon into the distance to a point when the conflict ceases. Reparation is about laying to rest how we feel about what has happened, and making amends or reconciliation in a fitting manner. It is not about victory, because just as with a real life conflict, the cost is often high and suffering too great to be celebrated when it ends. Also we do not know what the future holds one way or another. That is particularly why I chose the term reparation, because often the ending of a conflict is replete with a range of emotions of which the very least is happinesss or triumph. Instead recovery and mental illness are characterized by hope. Hope suggests a sense of relief, cautious optimism and the sense that we are still in and able to experience this life.

In recovery it is necessary to identify reliable means of support that have served us well before. Often these are personal, unique and situation-specific, and there is no guarantee that the same ones that worked before will always be effective. For example, the person's issues might have changed and there may be different features or reasons for the problems on this occasion, or it may simply be that what worked before is no longer effective. So, when finding methods to help us in recovery, we might look at (see Figure 9.1):

- What normally works?
- What does this add?
- Why might it be reliable again?

Answering these three questions might mean that the intervention we are considering could be useful but also that options that used to but which might not work now can be ruled out before we go to the trouble of trying them. Through this approach we may avoid ritualistic practice, acting out of habit, or making mistaken assumptions.

Figure 9.1 Finding methods for recovery

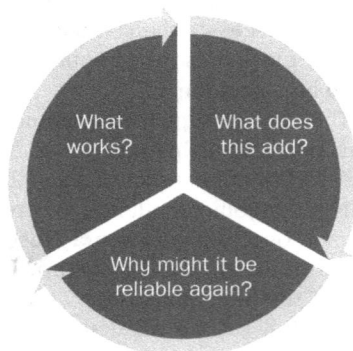

> **Exercise**
>
> Think back again to the above exercise on the 'parachute jump'. Once you had completed the challenge, were you surprised at just how easy it was? Was the hardest part not the challenge but overcoming the fear? Often the most significant steps forward that we make or the greatest progress is achieved more readily than we might expect.

Risk, rapport and reparation

A recovery-based approach can be promoted by the 3Rs. These are:

- *Risk*: Within the culture of the NHS there is a strong aversion to risk, with a preference for cautious and defensive practice and unpredictable or challenging situations, while commonplace, being regarded with anxiety and alarm. In turn, this can lead to service users being treated with suspicion, and stereotyping and labelling to occur (see Chapter 4, but also the example in Case Study 9.1 of Jodi). Practice that is consistent with recovery regards risk as something that needs to be recognized: it is a part of everyday life in acute mental health settings. This does not mean becoming complacent. Instead we need to be vigilant and assess and quantify risk where it is apparent. In this sense a balance is achieved between care and risk management that emphasizes the therapeutic relationship.
- *Rapport* contributes towards recovery in any setting, whether this is secure inpatient care, or between the mental health nurse and service user in the community. Recovery depends on the engagement, and sense of trust and investment in the therapeutic relationship. This does not necessarily mean that we have to know another person well, but it is important to feel a sense of engagement, believe in them and to feel motivated by them. Underlying the interaction with the service user is a sense of regard and commitment. As a mental health nurse, we need to ask ourselves, 'Do I have hope for this person?' The person in crisis, or with a severe and enduring mental health issue, is in an ongoing struggle with their mental health. They may experience repeated setbacks and reversals, and at times feel desolate. It is essential that we offer support and do not reinforce doubt.
- *Reparation* is a term that means to repair any damage done or to make recompense. When discussing the process of negotiations and settlement at the end of long, seemingly endless wars, it is noticeable that there is often a surprising lack of recrimination. Perhaps this is due to the exhaustion of the combatants. The relevance to mental health is that all crises, no matter how tumultuous, end at some point. War or conflict can be compared with the experience of mental illness. In my view, reparation in mental health means the terms upon which we resume life after the crisis. Reparation is the process whereby the person finds meaning and a way of overcoming, or coming

to terms with the loss(es) they may have experienced both emotionally as well as materially as a result of the illness. In reparation the person may say sorry to those they feel that they need to, or repair any damage that might have been caused, and make recompense but never need to accept blame simply for having a mental illness to begin with.

On a personal level, reparation refers to how the person now sees themselves in the light of the aftermath. Often this is complex and can be hard to describe in terms of one emotion. It may change from day to day, or depending on the person's mood. The incidence of relapse and repeated episodes of mental ill-health is extremely high for all mental health problems and some more than others (Gillespie, 2010; MHF, 2007; Rodgers et al., 2012). Therefore, reparation can mean restoration, and be helpful in identifying measures for relapse prevention, and tools that the service user has at their disposal. This involves the mental health nurse developing a sense of recovery that naturally flows into the post-acute phase of care and considering their mental health and well-being in the longer term. However, it will also mean that the service we provide is more cohesive and perceives mental health nursing more broadly and flexibly.

In the example in Case Study 9.1 that follows, we trace the evidence of the 3Rs and identify how they help in positively moving Jodie's care forward.

Case Study 9.1 Jodie

Jodi is 20 years old and has a loving and supportive family. After completing her compulsory education Jodi was not sure what she wanted to do and after working in numerous part-time jobs decided to go to university and move away from home. Jodi found it dificult living away from home, though, and struggled to make new friends. She went to see her GP who prescribed her anti-depressant medication. Recently her relationship with her boyfriend ended and she has failed her end-of-year exams. Jodi drank a large amount of alcohol, overdosed on tablets and self-harmed by cutting her wrists with a blade. After attending Accident and Emergency (A&E) and then spending some time on the Medical Assessment Unit (MAU) until her physical health stabilized, she was admitted as an informal patient to an open acute unit. Initially she was placed on general observation but was found cutting her arms, and disclosed that she had been habitually harming herself in this way. Jodi's observation levels were increased so she was within sight of a mental health nurse at all times and she was advised not to leave the unit.

In discussion with a member of staff Jodi said that the incident that led to her admission had not been a deliberate attempt to end her life. She said she had felt very low and desperate in the moment and the act of self-harming had been due to the stress and sense of self-doubt and uncertainty she was feeling.

Jodi felt that before coming into hospital her drinking and self-harm had been getting out of control. She said that she drinks to blot out difficult thoughts. On meeting her boyfriend she had kept these issues a secret, but as the term wore on and she became more homesick and then failed her exams, it became impossible to hide her distress. Jodie feels that seeing who she really is has put her boyfriend off, and led to him ending their relationship.

In a team meeting during handover it became apparent that there are two views among staff, both of which are quite strongly held views. One group regards Jodie as a 'typical late adolescent in crisis'. They see her as fully aware of her behaviour, highly capable and carefully calculating the risks she takes so they are not fatal. Consequently, there is a feeling of resentment towards her. In contrast, other members of the team feel more empathic. While accepting Jodi is highly articulate and cognitively mature, they feel that nevertheless she struggles emotionally with managing her responses to the issues that she is currently experiencing.

Q: Have you seen similar discussions in clinical areas on placement?

A: There is a danger that with regard to the first group of staff, Jodi may become stigmatized and labelled and her behaviours seen in isolation and not in their context (see Chapter 4). This might reduce the capacity of the staff to be able to empathize with Jodi due to suspicion over her motives. This may lead staff to be cautious and guarded when working with her. Jodi may be seen in terms of the risk that she represents, and the reasons for this not fully appreciated, which significantly limits the opportunity to work with her therapeutically.

An alternative view, held by the other group of staff, is that what we regard as risk in clinical settings is often the culmination of a series of factors over time. This accumulation of stressors can lead to a situation in which the individual responds in a manner that is dangerous to themselves or others, seeing no other option at this time. In other words, their capacity to cope has been exhausted. Often the factor leading to this event may seem to be innocuous, and the person's reaction can seem to be puzzling or to occur 'out of the blue'. In these circumstances it is essential to see the episode in the wider context of the circumstances of the service user's life. Zubin and Spring (1977) describe the stress-vulnerability model, whereby there is a relationship between stress factors, the individual's predisposing vulnerability and their overall capacity to cope. Enduring highly adverse circumstances over a sustained period of time exhausts the person's capacity to cope until their ability to manage is exhausted and a crisis occurs. Seen in terms of this model, when subjected to a range of stressors over a period of time, Jodi's coping mechanisms of drinking and self-harming became much more intense and she lapsed into crisis.

In order to fully understand risk, it is necessary to appreciate the context within which it occurs. Yet this is not always possible in acute settings where only the consequences of behaviours are evident. Both views have consequences not only for how we perceive risk, but also for the influence this then has upon the therapeutic rapport we are able to develop with the person.

Q: What are the potential consequences of the staff opinions on their therapeutic rapport with Jodi?

A: Where the staff resent Jodi, while this might not be apparent in what they say, it is likely to be evident in a whole range of subtle phenomena, from body language and facial expressions through to their possible reluctance to spend time with Jodi and a general manner of lacking interest in her well-being. These factors will have knock-on effects in terms of the ability of the staff to move Jodi's care forward in a positive manner. In contrast, the staff feel empathic towards Jodi are likely to be more willing and positive in their manner. They are also likely to help her to see a sense of purpose, and optimism for her future. In short, they are likely to be more inclined to 'be there' for her in a way that the first group of staff are not, which increases the likelihood that a productive therapeutic relationship can develop. Often these subtle behaviours can be pivotal in determining whether the service user engages with the mental health services or not. Also, the way in which negative attitudes such as those of the first group of staff are expressed, while perhaps seeming insignificant, can over time become ingrained and endemic within an organization, and become prevalent in the form of institutional discrimination whether against certain diagnoses, or other features such as race, as in the case of, for example, David Rocky Bennett (Norfolk, Suffolk and Cambridgeshire Strategic Health Authority, 2003).

To ensure Jodi's safety, based on the level of risk she presented, it is a good use of resources to place her on close observations. This situation can often feel claustrophobic for the service user, as they lose their privacy. However, if the person is in crisis and in a very changeable mental state, they may well feel unable to maintain their own safety. The constant presence of staff may serve as a source of reassurance and support at such times. Ultimately, it is Jodi's choice whether or not to engage therapeutically. The close physical proximity she has with the nursing staff means there is significant potential for the attitude of the staff to exert an influence upon the therapeutic relationship that unfolds.

The transition from risk to rapport

Rapport is the basis of a sound therapeutic relationship with the service user. A rapport can be understood as a cordial relationship in which those involved have a mutual appreciation of one another's ideas and feelings, and can communicate (Jenkins and Elliott, 2004). It might be felt that the process of close observation could limit the potential for an open therapeutic relationship. Fortunately, this is not necessarily so. While the therapeutic relationship is imposed upon Jodi to a large extent, nevertheless there are choices as to what happens next and the focus of the relationship is on her care and well-being. This could be seen as a sound basis for developing a therapeutic rapport. In other cases, though, where, for example, there is a possibility of aggression from the service user, working to de-escalate aggressive situations offering choice and removing confrontation are essential. When developing a therapeutic rapport, optimizing the service user's scope for choice and assuming independence is essential.

During the close observations, the focus of the therapeutic rapport was to negotiate towards a goal of Jodi being able to regain independence, initially through maintaining her own safety. On being placed on close observation, Jodi's mood was very subdued and low to begin with, but as time wore on she engaged well with some members of the ward team and discussed her situation quite openly.

Often a rapport can be developed by carrying out activities with the service user, ranging from mealtimes through to everyday activities concerning life. Frequently, the most therapeutic conversations occur when the person is not consciously focused upon their thoughts and feelings. Being on close observation provides plenty of opportunities for everyday activities to become therapeutic, and a natural means of engaging with the service user.

With the support of staff, Jodi completed the Recovery Star (see below). The Recovery Star consists of 10 areas that are scored from 1–10 but these are paired in stages (see Table 9.1).

Table 9.1 Scoring ladder for the Recovery Star

Score	Stage	Features
9–10	**Self-reliance**	New behaviours are established and function well, and the service user needs less help. At the top of the scale the service user can function positively in terms of their own needs, and in relation to others around them, and knows where to access help and support when required
7–8	**Learning**	Through the process of trial and error setbacks and reversals are encountered but overcome. As a result of this process the service user gains a better idea of what works in moving forward and making positive progress. Yet there is still an emphasis on working with services and talking things through and gaining support
5–6	**Believing**	The service user believes that positive change is possible and is gaining confidence in making these steps and doing things differently
3–4	**Accepting help**	The service user accepts there is a problem, but perhaps is not confident of making a change, or where there is change, it is unlikely to be sustained without support
1–2	**Stuck**	The service user is stuck, and perhaps not accepting that there is a problem, unable to believe that there is anyone who might be able to help but perhaps with occasional feelings of wishing to change

Source: MacKeith and Burns (2011).

The 10 areas of the Recovery Star are:

- *Managing mental health*: Within the traditional approach medication or symptoms may be considered instead. This area looks at how well the person can lead their life in a way that is not limited by mental illness.
- *Physical health and self-care*: '. . . taking care of your physical health, keeping clean, how you present yourself, being able to deal with stress and knowing how to keep yourself feeling well' (MacKeith and Burns, 2011: 6).
- *Living skills*: These include being able to live independently and do cleaning, shopping and cooking and getting on with neighbours and visitors.
- *Social networks*: Being a part of the community in terms of engaging with others and in activities.
- *Work*: Whether in a paid or voluntary capacity but also the education and training needed to get a desired job and knowing what it is that you want to do.
- *Relationships*: Particularly with regard to the person closest to you and whether you want that relationship to be better and closer or if you do not have a close relationship but would like one.
- *Addictive behaviour*: In terms of awareness of addictive behaviour and the harm to self or others. These include alcohol, substance misuse, eating, gambling or shopping.
- *Responsibilities*: Includes paying rent, relating to others we live alongside and abiding by the law.
- *Identity and self-esteem*: Who the person is and their strengths and weaknesses and, if applicable, their cultural, religious and spiritual identity.
- *Trust and hope*: Belief in a positive future and the ability to feel able to trust others.

On completing the Recovery Star (see Figure 9.2), Jodi was surprised at how much it made her reflect on her own responsibilities and the way in which she understood them.

Exercise

Look at the description of the areas of the Recovery Star above.

- How do you think Jodi might score and in what areas might she feel she has the most problem?
- Discuss this with a classmate or friend and compare your scores. Was there a significant difference?
- Which areas of the Recovery Star did you find more or less difficult to apply and why?

Figure 9.2 The Recovery Star

Source: http://www.recoverywirral.com/wordpress/wp-content/uploads/recoveryStar.jpg (MacKeith and Burns, 2011).

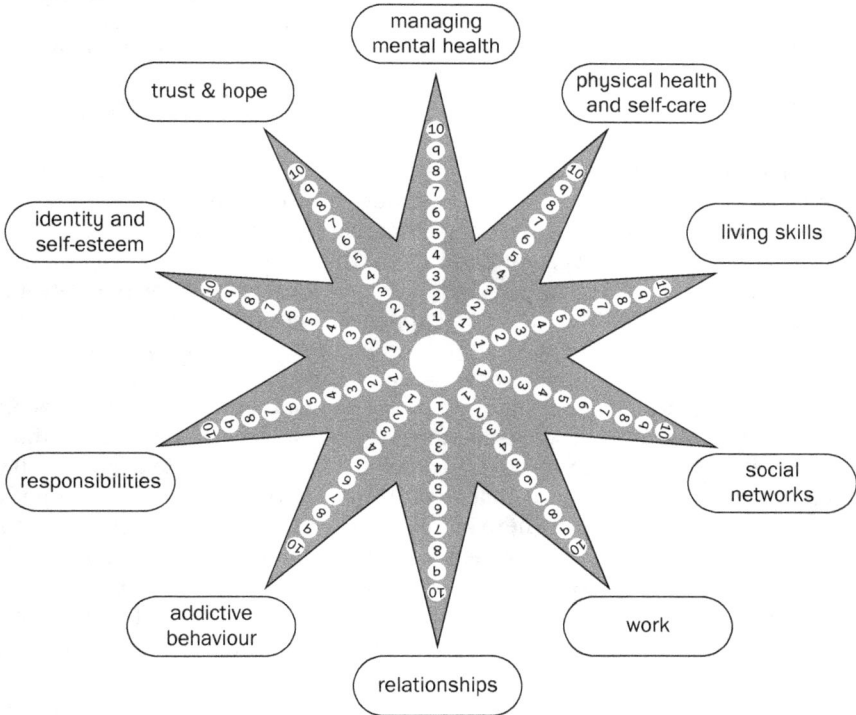

Case Study 9.1   Jodi (continued)

After just under a week Jodi's mood seemed to lift for a consistent period of time, and following discussions between the multidisciplinary team (MDT) and Jodi, it was agreed to lower the level of observations. In traditional approaches, decisions regarding observation levels are often made without consultation with the service user. Consulting the service user is a collaborative practice, and promotes empowerment. It means that the service user is involved in the decision-making process, and enabled to be aware of how their decisions influence their care. In this sense, working with risk becomes a therapeutic process in which the service user is jointly involved in working towards regaining independence with the support of the mental health team. This represents meaningful recovery.

Mindfulness

Jodi particularly found the mindfulness sessions held on the ward to be useful. Mindfulness is based on an Eastern, esoteric approach to life, the modern version of which is credited as having been pioneered by Jon Kabat Zinn (1990/2013) and proceeds on the basis of 'living in the moment'. Williams and Penman's text of 2011, *Mindfulness: A Practical Guide to Finding Peace in a Frantic World*, is a key source in providing a useful programme by which to learn this method.

To understand mindfulness, it helps to consider how we experience time. Often this is seen as being linear (see Figure 9.3) with the past, present and future all being a way of measuring the passing seconds, minutes and hours tracing a uniform and consistent pattern into the future.

This is not the case, however, as we experience the states of the past, present and future differently. The past has happened, and although irretrievable is documented, and stored away in our minds. It is remembered to the extent that any of us can recall and relive events. We have a wealth of memories and recollections, some of which are easily remembered, and others that are more deeply submerged within our consciousness. Have you ever remembered something that you thought you had forgotten? The philosopher Martin Heidegger (2003) suggests that a more accurate conceptualization of time is that we constantly live in the present, as that is where our existence at any particular point is situated. Yet at the same time the present instantly becomes the past, and is gone, therefore the present in which we live is the most important aspect of these past, present and future states of time. Yet it is also the most brief and fleeting moment, because as we focus on a moment, it instantly becomes the past. Meanwhile the future is there to be seen. The immediate future forms the next instant of time that we experience. In Figure 9.4 this notion of time is depicted as intermeshing gears, whereby the past has led us to the present, which, in turn, transports us to the future. Figure 9.4 shows that the present is the largest of the cogs as it is the one that we are most aware of, yet ironically it inhabits the least actual amount of time.

Mindfulness represents a way we can better fit our experience and perceptions within the nature of time by living fully and entirely in the present. Mindfulness proceeds on the basis that often our experience of the present is clouded

Figure 9.3 A linear concept of time

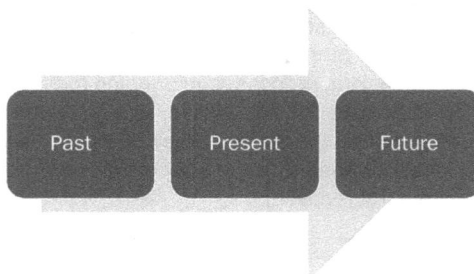

Figure 9.4 The passing of time

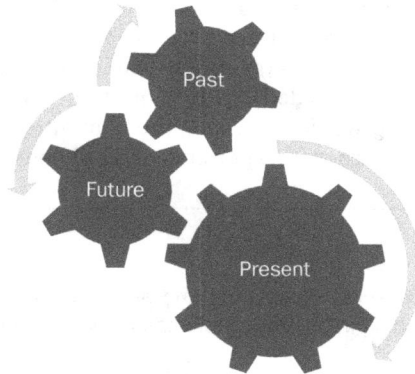

Figure 9.5 The mindfulness and past-present-future continuum

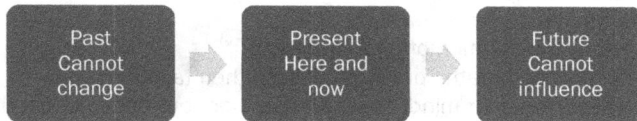

by so many preoccupations and other concerns and burdens. In mindfulness the emphasis is on living within and being in the present. Moments of reflection and concentration and focusing on ourselves and our bodies and surroundings can lead to an intense appreciation of even very small and minute aspects of our lives. Yet these are of immense personal value and meaning. These experiences are sometimes captured in a moment, yet this brief capsule of time may seem to be far longer than the actual duration due to the quality of the experience. The more we devote ourselves to developing skills of living within the moment, the more we appreciate and value life.

Mindfulness emphasizes paying attention, in a non-judgemental way, to the 'here and now'. It uses techniques that encourage us to listen and become attuned to our body, and in particular our breathing. This can help us to change the focus of our attention: instead of worrying about our concerns from the past and future, we are absorbed in the present moment. If we refer back to the beginning of the chapter, and the example of the activity that you were afraid of, how much did it affect the situation that you thought about it in advance of the event? Often events that we feel apprehensive about provoke anxious thoughts within us, and consequently our fears multiply. As Figure 9.5 demonstrates, mindfulness encourages us to exist in the present and forget about the future and the past. If we stop worrying so much about them, we might achieve more in the present unencumbered by what we cannot change.

Mindfulness encourages us to focus our attention in the present, and to stop worrying about events that we cannot change or influence, whether in the future or past. Yet this is not to suggest that the past or future are meaningless or have no implications for the present, just that often we need to stop and exist in the here and now. Yet this is a skill, and requires a lot of practice for most of us. If we struggle with anxiety or are prone to rumination, it may seem even more challenging to 'let thoughts go' rather than engaging with them. Mindfulness requires commitment and dedication in order for us to become competent. It needs to be something we do regularly, are committed to, and is something that requires practice in order to experience the full benefit.

Exercise

Check that you have some spare time and are in a comfortable place away from distractions and sit in a comfortable chair away from any noise or music and put away your phone.

- Close your eyes and focus on your breathing.
- Breathe at a steady and normal rate.
- Let your breathing happen naturally.
- Feel the depth of your breath.
- Be aware of the duration of your breathing.
- Do not count the breaths or length of time they take.
- If thoughts enter your mind, acknowledge them but don't get caught up in them – observe them as though from a distance, like an image on a cinema screen.
- Try this for five minutes.

Adapted from Williams and Penman (2011)

Now, think about how you feel:

- refreshed;
- a bit more alert;
- more lively;
- happy;
- more in the here and now;
- other feeling.

If you struggled to relax, do not be hard on yourself. Ironically, relaxing is hard work, and takes practice and time to learn. Relaxing in this way on a regular basis becomes easier the more you do it and with practice. Follow the guidance above, or a variation of it on a regular basis and you will feel more relaxed. Once you have been able to listen to your breathing, focus on your body. Progressive Muscle Relaxation (Anxiety BC, 2016) is a useful way of relaxing using this method. Alternatively, you might carry out a mental body scan, focusing on your body one section at a time from your head and neck to each of your shoulders and chest all the way down to your toes to identify and relieve tensions and tightness and to feel more relaxed physically and mentally.

We are aware of far more than we might think. It is often the case that our attention is drawn to what we think we need to focus upon, what we need to do for our work role, or what we are told to pay attention to, as opposed to what is actually catching our attention. In spite of being focused on the present, once you start practising mindfulness these techniques might sharpen your alertness. You may find that when reflecting at other times than engaged specifically in mindfulness, you remember events in the past more clearly than you did before, and other aspects of these experiences become more apparent. Smells, sensations, feelings and other sensory stimuli are also powerfully evocative, and you may find these are triggered more frequently. You may remember more. And a wider variety of events than you ever realized that you did. Essentially, mindfulness and concentrating on living in the present promote quality of life, and add depth to experience.

Mindfulness ought not to be confused with distraction or hypnosis, but instead refers to consciously living in the moment. It seems like a simple concept but it does take time and practice to develop and will improve with training. Living in the present can also be achieved by other methods, such as colouring patterns, wordsearches, crosswords, Soduko or other word games.

Reparation

Reparation is giving back, repaying or making recompense but also restoring who we are. Mary Ellen Copeland's WRAP (see Chapter 11) discusses the need to redress losses that may have occurred in the crisis period; whether these are emotional, psychological, physical or financial. For example, where the person has carried out self-harm, there may be long-term consequences that need to be dealt with, such as physical damage or impairments to health. Where the person has spent a significant amount of money when unwell, arrangements may need to be made to pay this back, or arrange for repayments, and there is quite literally a need to make recompense. Restoration may occur in terms of re-establishing who we are, taking on old responsibilities and becoming who we are again in relationships we may have neglected or allowed to lapse during the crisis. The notions of recompense and restoration are flexible and will apply differently in different situations. However, it is an important principle that the service user does not experience recrimination.

For example, in the Case Study of Andy in Chapter 8, it is difficult though necessary to overcome self-blame and labelling as a result of having a mental health problem, while Denise may feel resentful and angry towards Andy. She may experience problems within the relationship through feeling unexpressed resentment towards Andy that may become apparent in other ways. It may be necessary for Andy and Denise to seek counselling as a couple if they feel that there are underlying and residual issues that need to be dealt with. Often people with mental health issues experience strains, and even the loss of close personal relationships as a result of mental illness. Essentially, reparation and the immediate post-crisis phase of illness about resumption, and how we carry on with life (see Figure 9.6).

Reparation involves the notion that mental illness may be a part of the person's life on an ongoing basis and a recurrent feature. Such notions conflict

Figure 9.6 Aspects of reparation

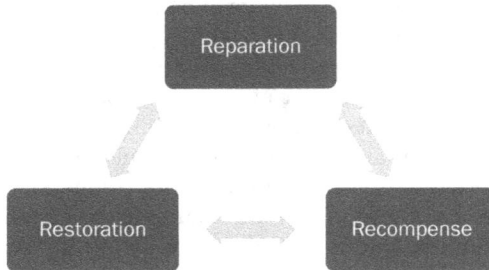

with the traditional approach to mental health that focuses on clinical out-comes ('getting well') as the main measure of improvement. While the whole point of service intervention is for the person's level of distress to reduce, and their crisis to dissipate, there are other factors to consider. Sometimes recovery means returning to the circumstances that led the person to experience crisis in the first place. However, the situation may be experienced differently as the person learns from their experience and gains in self-knowledge and the ability to organize their life, know themselves more, and acquires further coping skills. Part of this process is the discovery of effective self-management strategies and methods of building resilience. This could be seen as individual action research, or the development of a personalized evidence-based approach on the part of the service user. Recovery is often seen as working with what we have at the time, and listening to ourselves to ensure that new knowledge is continually woven into our approach. This involves unflinching honesty and integrity, and also a sense of commitment and purpose. Often the ability to engage in this process stems not so much from confidence as losing the sense of fear.

Once again, if we recall the exercise at the start of this chapter, we are often held back by fear. It can stop us achieving what we really aspire to, and per-haps the most significant issue that we need to address is to develop a new relationship to fear. Instead of avoiding fear, we need to face it, confront it, and to learn new ways to manage its effects on us (Jeffers, 2011). Similarly, in our professional role as a mental health nurse, we can encourage service users to cultivate a sense of self-awareness, which will enhance personal development. Confidence grows through becoming aware of our strengths, skills and identity but also having the courage to recognize our fears and confront them.

Towards the end of Jodi's inpatient admission, she became calmer in mood and more settled. Even though the duration of her inpatient stay was brief (just 2–3 weeks), for Jodi this introduced a major change in her view of life. Jodi said that she felt immensely guilty and ashamed at having taken the over-dose and carrying out the self-harm. Guilt or shame is a common experience following a crisis, and represents a part of the process of reconciling ourselves with the experiences we undergo. This illustrates the notion of reparation, and is a common feature of recovery from substance misuse, addiction and coming to terms with the feelings that lead to self-harming behaviour. Too often people with mental health problems undergo self-stigmatization and experience self-loathing and blame, and this compounds their already lacking sense of self-worth as a result of not experiencing reconciliation with what has happened.

Sometimes a sense of euphoria also occurs. If we think back to the exercise at the beginning of the chapter, it is sometimes invigorating to overcome a challenge and emerge from a crisis that has at times felt overwhelming and that can lead to a similar energy boost. This needs to be managed carefully to prevent there being a subsequent dip in mood in the immediate post-treatment aftermath when life returns to normal and the euphoria fades.

Jodi has learned some valuable lessons about herself. She has decided not to return to her university course, choosing to take some time to reflect on her ambitions, and feels that she will cope better with stressful situations in the future. In moving forward the MDT and Jodi felt that she might benefit from dialectical behavioural therapy (DBT) and support with emotional regulation and anxiety management.

Conclusion

In this chapter we have discussed practical approaches to recovery largely through the Case Study of Jodi. We discussed recovery in terms of the 3Rs of Risk, Rapport and Reparation. How we perceive risk has important consequences for the therapeutic rapport. It helps to view it as part of the therapeutic role of the mental health nurse consistent with recovery and not purely from the perspective of just risk as one isolated function of the mental health nurse's role. We then discussed the Recovery Star, which has emerged as an influential and popular tool within a range of different mental health services and is adaptable and service user-focused. The Recovery Star performs an important role in empowering the service user in determining where they are situated at any particular time and where and how they wish to make progress. We also considered mindfulness. This is widely used and highly effective in all areas of mental health nursing. Yet in order to be effective, mindfulness needs to be actively practised within our lives as well, so that we can know its benefits and discuss it meaningfully with service users, as opposed to just recommending it. The discussion then moved on to look at reparation. Due to the strikingly high rates of relapse for numerous mental health issues, planning ahead and using what is learned from the experience of crisis are essential. In the chapters that follow in Section 3 of the book, we look at other models of recovery that also emphasize the role of learning from the experience of mental health problems.

Section 3

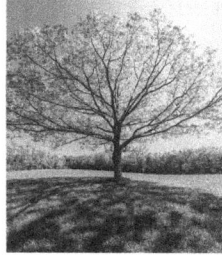

Models of recovery

10 Models of recovery

Kike Abioye

Introduction

We all go through life with some beliefs about what our experience means. It seems that this is often what lends purpose to our life and gives a point to our existence. Within mental health nursing, it is essential to develop a personal vision of recovery that is genuine and real, and incorporate it into our practice. So far in this book we have looked at our values and how these relate to the principles of the profession of mental health nursing. We have also discussed how we reflect upon our experiences to make recovery an everyday aspect of our practice. Building on this understanding, we now look at mental health nursing-focused models of recovery.

Models reflect beliefs about the nature of health problems, the purpose and role of nursing and how we engage and collaborate with service users. In this chapter we look at the major mental health nursing-focused models that use a recovery-based approach. We begin by thinking about what defines a model of nursing. Then we will explain Barker's (2003) Tidal Model. In the second part of the chapter we move on to look at Repper and Perkins' (2003) Psychosocial Model.

By the end of this chapter readers will have:

- an understanding of mental health-focused nursing models;
- a practical understanding of the Tidal Model;
- a practical perspective of Repper and Perkins' Psychosocial Model.

What are models?

Models became prominent from the 1980s onwards with the movement of nursing into higher education (Pearson et al., 2005). It was felt that the increasing emphasis on nursing theory required the support of a conceptual basis to justify practice. Essentially, like recovery, nursing models are a philosophy. They reflect a consistent interconnected and thematically linked set of beliefs about how health functions. But alongside this there is an understanding of what nursing is, how it is delivered and how we can know whether it is effective.

There are numerous different models, including: Neuman, Orem, Parse, Peplau and Roper et al. (Forchuk, 1993; Hartweg, 1991; Neuman, 1995; Nurseslabs, 2016; Nursing Theory, 2016). Most are characterized by having been developed in bygone decades by influential nursing practitioners with many years' experience. Models have a range of features and characteristics, and some of the various definitions and understandings are listed in the following box.

Models of nursing

There are different definitions and understandings of models. Here are some of them:

- Models represent collections of theories, beliefs and knowledge (Wrycraft, 2009).
- Models can also be seen as conceptual tools that help us take complex information, organize it and place it into perspective (McKenna, 1997, 2014; McKenna and Slevin, 2008).
- Models can be represented in a variety of forms, ranging from words, pictures, diagrams, flow charts or graphs (Chinn and Kramer, 2008).
- A model is a multidimensional concept that defines the way in which healthcare services are delivered (McAllister and Moyle, 2008).
- Models are like blueprints that provide guidance for the planning and the delivery of nursing care in mental health practice (Cutcliffe et al., 2010).
- A model of healthcare has a distinct framework and design; a theoretical basis and defined standards; evidence-based practices; and measurable outcomes or key performance indicators (Davidson et al., 2006).

Exercise

Now refer back to the above definitions of nursing models, and read them all through again. Select just one and write down how it helps the delivery of mental health nursing in practice. Also why did you choose that definition of a model above the others? Which features stand out for you and why?

Unfortunately in recent decades there have not been too many newer nursing models. Those discussed in this chapter date from the early to mid-2000s, yet compared to many others are quite modern. Perhaps this reflects the change in nursing in recent years with a greater emphasis on pace, the performance of tasks and saving costs in a high-demand setting. Arguably, nursing knowledge has focused more on technology and achieving tasks as opposed to the more conceptual and philosophical meanings on which the profession rests. While nurses may now be performing a wider range of more complex roles, this is at the expense of creating a workforce that can use deeper underlying knowledge and autonomous problem-solving skills.

Certainly within nursing education, there is less inclination to specifically teach and assess students' understanding of nursing models than in previous eras. In spite of this, Wrycraft (2009) and Pryjmachuk (2011) suggest that nursing models still have relevance in informing and assisting mental health nurses in working with service users. Nursing models also provide reasons why we carry out actions and allow us to work within an overall consistent approach. The move away from models is disappointing, and perhaps with a regrettable consequence that values, principles and recovery are not more prominent in practice.

There are two especially popular models within mental health nursing. These are the Tidal Model of Barker and Buchanan-Barker (2005) and the Psychosocial Model of Repper and Perkins (2003). They were developed in mental health settings and wholly centred on the person's understanding of health. Both models proceed from a philosophy of recovery, considering what health means for the person physically, psychologically and socially, regardless of the clinical symptoms of mental health problems.

The Tidal Model

The Tidal Model is a recovery-based approach that values the language of service users to describe their experience (Barker and Buchanan-Barker, 2005). The model does not pathologize mental health issues as medical problems, but instead sees them in a much wider context as a human experience with the service user taking the responsibility for change (Stevenson and Fletcher, 2002). At the root of the Tidal Model is Hildegard Peplau's theory of interpersonal relations and transactions through empowerment (Barker, 2001; Jones, 1996; Peplau, 1988). Consistent with Peplau, the Tidal Model seeks to develop a constructive therapeutic relationship between the service user and nurse. This allows for the exploration of the service user's circumstance within a caring environment that promotes growth (Barker, 2001).

An important departure from many other models that focus on deficits is that the Tidal Model emphasizes the recognition of personal strengths, skills and attributes. It was developed as a result of a five-year research study undertaken at the University of Newcastle and is the first mental health recovery-focused model jointly developed by nurses and service users (Buchanan-Barker and Barker, 2008). The title of 'Tidal' was chosen to reflect the fluid, ever-changing and unpredictable nature of human experience, yet other language that is also used within the model is also based on a maritime theme. For example: 'washed up', 'swimming against the tide', 'drowning' and 'all at sea' (Barker, 2003; Barker and Buchanan-Barker, 2005; Stevenson and Fletcher, 2002). There is an apt resonance between the experience of being shipwrecked and lost at sea and the turmoil of individuals in a crisis with their mental health.

The tidal domains within the nursing care/process

The Tidal Model comprises three interrelated domains of assessment and intervention. These are the 'Self', the 'World' and 'Others'. Figure 10.1 demonstrates how each of the domains represents a dimension of the person's being and identity. The domains represent the separate yet interconnected dimensions of the person's life, and are the metaphorical settings representing the individual's life story (Barker and Buchanan-Barker, 2005). The aim of the nursing assessment is to develop a better understanding of the influences on the individual from each of the domains and how interventions within each of these areas will help with problems of living.

The 'Self' domain

Where the person is, for example, experiencing psychosis or schizophrenia, they may struggle to identify what their thoughts are and the products of their own mind and the phenomena produced externally to them. Alternatively, difficult feelings such as guilt and shame may lead the person to deny or find it hard to accept aspects themselves. While in depression, low self-esteem may lead the person not to want to think about themselves. Alternatively, people with some types of personality disorder may be narcissistic, and have an emphasis on their own interests at the expense of others. As this domain pertains to the person's sense of themselves, there are implications for their potential to remain safe, and it is essential to conduct a risk assessment, and

Figure 10.1 Domains of the Tidal Model

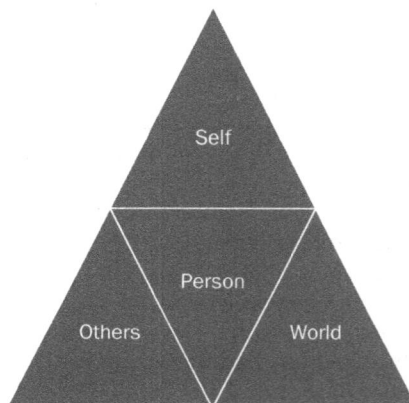

develop a person-centred personal security plan (Barker and Buchanan-Barker, 2005). The plan identifies the personal and interpersonal resources and considers any threat posed to personal security or that of others (Barker and Buchanan-Barker, 2005).

The 'World' domain

The 'World' domain refers to the person's way of engaging with their environment. It relates to storytelling, and is facilitated through holistic assessment and in-depth conversation (Barker and Buchanan-Barker, 2005). Within this view we may deploy a narrative approach (Coad and Wrycraft, 2015). Within this understanding people form a personal understanding of their life. For example, I worked with people with dementia in inpatient settings and often a person would say they needed to go home to make tea for their children or to put them to bed. Often this was not an isolated comment but part of a well-developed set of ideas and apparently a candid belief that the person was still looking after their young children. All of this in spite of their children having long since grown up and having children of their own and the person themselves now being in older age. The point of this example is that often we develop explanations for our situation. Yet these are more than just reasons. They consist of experiences and memories.

In Chapter 9 we discussed the past. This is more than just what has happened to us before and consigned to history. Instead our past forms a valuable repository of experiences that we can often draw upon. For example, in the case of a person who is experiencing dementia, in their past they may have been a busy and responsible parent and felt love, valued, rewarded and fulfilled. In their current reality they may have difficulty communicating and understanding the reality around them and feel disempowered. In some cases it may be assumed that this is a feature of their dementia and the result of confusion or they may be hallucinating. Yet, from a narrative perspective, the fact that the person repeatedly returns to these experiences and different aspects rather than confusion suggests that there is a consistent story and this phenomenon has a different cause.

A narrative view may instead suggest that the person immerses themselves in a former contented phase of their life as a means of compensating for their current difficulties and gaining reassurance but also of making sense of the present. In this way stories help us to make sense of situations. Narrative theory also suggests that we try and make sense of our reality. In the case of a person with schizophrenia, often the voices that are experienced form part of an elaborate system of ideas that often do not seem to be based in reality yet have a tenuous link to events in the person's life. When working with service users in this situation, it helps to understand the person's narrative. It also helps to avoid agreeing with the person that what they are saying is factually correct. However, being willing to listen to the service user's story helps in developing a functional therapeutic rapport and crucially builds trust and encourages engagement. This is especially helpful where the person is experiencing paranoia. The aim is to help the individual narrate the story of what has happened with a view to discussing and identifying what could address any problems (Barker and Buchanan-Barker, 2005).

The 'Others' domain

The 'Others' domain allows the person to act out their life story together with others. This is evident in how the service user and others are mutually influential through social encounters (Barker and Buchanan-Barker, 2005). The others domain generates one-to-one conversations focused on helping the person identify and discuss issues and problems, but also strengths and possible resources. From this basis the person can identify what they might do, or receive from others to begin to address the issues (Barker and Buchanan-Barker, 2005).

Exercise

- From what you have read so far about the Tidal Model, what are the challenges of implementing it in inpatient clinical settings?
- Consider which of the domains would come first when assessing a person in order to promote their recovery.

Central to the Tidal Model is collaboration that creates a platform to work with the individual through the remaining Tidal domains and processes (Barker and Buchanan-Barker, 2005; Centre of Excellence in Interdisciplinary Mental Health (CEIMH) and University of Birmingham and Birmingham and Solihull Mental Health (BSMHT), 2008). This is necessary to establish a therapeutic relationship that will enhance the recovery journey (Barker and Buchanan-Barker, 2006; CEIMH and BSMHT, 2008; Pryjmachuk, 2011). The Tidal Model embraces philosophical assumptions that are central to recovery-focused practice (Buchanan-Barker and Barker, 2006). These assumptions are equally specific about people, their experience of problems of living, and their capacity for change (Barker and Buchanan-Barker, 2005). A set of related values for the model have been developed from these assumptions, and these form the Tidal 10 commitments and the 20 competencies expected of the professionals working with individuals (Barker and Buchanan-Barker 2005). The commitments identify principles of the model in terms of being broad statements that demonstrate beliefs about the nature of the role of the nurse, and how we ought to be with service users. The competencies provide guidance for practice, demonstrating how the commitments might be carried out in practice. However, of course, these only represent guidance, and many other actions and interventions can be used that also meet the principles of the commitments.

The 10 commitments and the 20 competencies

Commitment 1: Value the voice: The Tidal Model helps people develop their unique narrative accounts into a formalized version of 'my story', through ensuring that all assessments and records of care are written in the person's own 'voice'.

Competency 1: Demonstrate the skilful capacity to actively listen to the service user's story.

Competency 2: Be committed to supporting the service user record their life story in their own words as part of the ongoing process of care in the first person singular.

Commitment 2: Respect the language: Using the individual's exact and unique language, statement of description of their needs. This represents the simplest, yet most powerful respect for the individual (Buchanan-Barker and Barker, 2008).

Competency 3: Assist the individual to express themselves in their own language by using the same phrases and words as the service user.

Competency 4: Help the person to express their understanding of particular experiences through the use of personal stories, anecdotes, similes or metaphors.

Commitment 3: Develop genuine curiosity: Genuineness and unflinching interest help the professional to know and understand the service user and gain a detailed account of their story. Curiosity provides a better understanding of features of the storyteller's mental health problem (Buchanan-Barker and Barker, 2008).

Competency 5: Display your interest in the individual's life story by asking for clarification on specific points and for further examples or details.

Competency 6: Be willing to help the individual relate their story at their own chosen pace and pattern.

Commitment 4: Become the apprentice: You are not likely to know an individual more than they know themselves. So patiently learn what they need from the individual who is an expert on their own life story; you can never know another person's experience (Buchanan-Barker and Barker, 2008; Szasz, 2000).

Competency 7: Develop the plan of care based on the expressed and collaboratively identified needs, wants or wishes of the service user.

Competency 8: Support the individual to identify specific problems of living, and what might need to be carried out to address the problems.

Commitment 5: Reveal personal wisdom: Over time and through their life the individual has developed a powerful storehouse of wisdom. In contemporary mental health, the individual's story is often framed by powerful metaphors, which convey the magnitude of their distress (Barker, 2003). Listening to, and hearing the service user's story expressed in their own language and terms, permits us to see the real person.

Competency 9: Assist the individual to identify and develop their awareness of personal strengths and weaknesses that will sustain the individual in their voyage of recovery (Buchanan-Barker and Barker, 2006).

Competency 10: Support the person to develop self-belief by promoting their ability to help themselves.

Commitment 6: Be transparent: Being involved in an individual's life story is a privilege that must be handled with respect and dignity. Be clear and transparent at all times. Help the individual understand what is being carried out and why by retaining their language and accuracy of description, and work in collaboration with the individual.

Competency 11: Aim to ensure that the person is aware, at all times, of the purpose of all processes of care.

Competency 12: Ensure that the individual is provided with copies of all assessment and care planning documents for their own reference.

Commitment 7: Use the available kit: The service user's story contains many examples of what has worked for them in the past, or beliefs about what may work for them in the future. These represent the primary tools that need to be used to unlock or build the story of recovery. The professional toolkit, commonly expressed through ideas such as evidence-based practice, describes what appears to have worked for other clients. Yet this should only be used if the client's available toolkit is lacking.

Competency 13: Help the service user to develop awareness of what works for or against them in relation to specific problems of living.

Competency 14: Display interest in identifying what the individual thinks specific people can or might be able to do to help them further in dealing with specific problems of living.

Commitment 8: Craft the step beyond: It helps to support the service user in envisioning moving forward. Crafting the step beyond emphasizes the relevance of working with the service user in their current situation to address what needs to happen for the service user's next step.

Competency 15: Support the service user to identify the kind of change that would represent a step in the direction of resolving or moving away from a specific problem of living.

Competency 16: Assist the service user to identify what needs to happen in the immediate future to enable them to make a 'positive step' in the direction of their desired goal.

Commitment 9: Give the gift of time: Time as often said is the midwife of change. There is nothing more valuable than giving time to listen to the service user, and become 'the apprentice'.

Competency 17: Ensure that the service user is aware that dedicated and constructive time is being given to addressing their specific needs.

Competency 18: Acknowledge the value of the time the service user gives to the process of assessment and care delivery.

Commitment 10: Know that change is possible: Change is inevitable because it is constant, and the truth is that nothing lasts.

Competency 19: Help the service user develop an awareness of how change is happening; knowledge could be used to steer them out of danger and distress back on to the course of reclamation and recovery through individual thoughts, feelings or action.

Competency 20: Help the service user develop awareness of how they, others or events have influenced the desired changes.

Exercise

- From reading about them above, reflect and write down in your own words how you would define each of the 10 commitments.
- Now read the commitments again and compare how your interpretation differs. Think about how your understanding is different, and what aspects do you emphasize?

Two people can witness an event happening and come away with entirely different perceptions of what has happened. Within the context of their lives, it can also mean something radically different as well. The Tidal Model emphasizes the individual's narrative account. Consistent with this individual and personal approach, the language that is used must be carefully chosen to portray the relevance of the narrative account with fidelity to the individual's intentions (CEIMH and BSMHT, 2008). The mental health nurse listens, hears and understands the service user's story from their perspective (CEIMH and BSMHT, 2008). In this part of the chapter, we have looked at an understanding of nursing models and the Tidal Model of recovery. Next we consider Repper and Perkins' (2003) Psychosocial Model.

Recovery and social inclusion: the Psychosocial Model

Mental health is a biopsychosocial phenomenon. This theory is widely credited as having begun with George Engel's seminal paper published in 1977. A biopsychosocial model regards health as consisting of biological, psychological and sociological aspects (see Figure 10.2). These are specific areas, yet they function by acting together in synthesis.

An implication of this notion is that for people with mental health issues not everything that appears to be biological is necessarily amenable to medical treatment. Psychological and sociological features of mental health problems can lead to biological features, whereas biological issues can also influence aspects of the person's psychological and sociological functioning. This seems to be self-evident. For example, if you live with constant back pain, which blights your life in every way, your mood may deteriorate. Your physical health then has a direct effect upon your mental health. How people experience health problems is a complex and multifaceted phenomenon. There are many different ways in which the biopsychosocial aspects of health can exert an influence on each other. For example, a person may experience low mood and this is expressed in the form of a physical health issue for which there seems to be no explanation.

The biopsychosocial theory of health and recovery are very compatible concepts. Understanding that health issues have complex causes also implies

Figure 10.2 Biopsychosocial concept of health

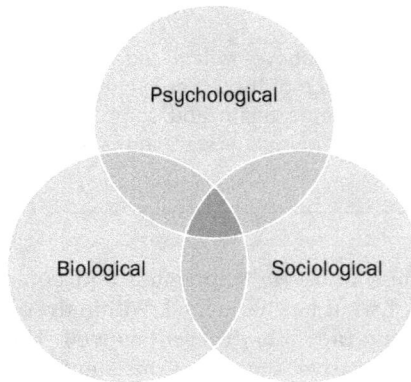

that the solutions and interventions will also often be individual and particular. The role of the mental health nurse is essential in developing a good therapeutic rapport with the service user towards facilitating recovery-focused care. Yet central to recovery is that the service user initiates the change and is empowered in the process.

Often people with mental health problems report that more disabling than the effects of their illness are the negative social impacts and the effects of exclusion and stigma. It takes more than medication and/or therapies for service users to recover their lives. When supporting the person during recovery in the community, it is necessary to work to create opportunities for social inclusion. Hence the need for a psychosocial model that emphasizes positive attributes, strengths and skills, rather than problems, diagnosis and dysfunction (Perkins and Repper, 2013).

Repper and Perkins' (2003) Psychosocial Model looks at how recovery-focused mental healthcare ought to be organized to facilitate and promote social inclusion. The Psychosocial Model aims to support individuals in accessing roles and relationships with significant others, as well as engaging in activities that are valuable to them. Their model has three components. These are: personal adaptation, access and inclusion, and developing hope-inspiring relationships. These three parts of the model interrelate and overlap as shown in Figure 10.3.

The stages of the model are not sequential. Instead, in order to make progress in each of these areas, there is a high level of synchronicity between the aspects. *Personal adaptation* pertains to using the person's resources for recovery. These include attributes such as confidence and self-belief, but also competencies, skills and aspirations for the future. This aspect of the model also involves supporting the person to understand and accept what has happened; and to gain some control over their mental health and life. *Access and inclusion* involves the resources that we need to live, for example, money, clothing, housing and utilities, household equipment and supplies and food. Yet also supporting the person in roles, relationships and activities, for example,

Figure 10.3 The Psychosocial Model
Source: Adapted from Repper and Perkins (2003).

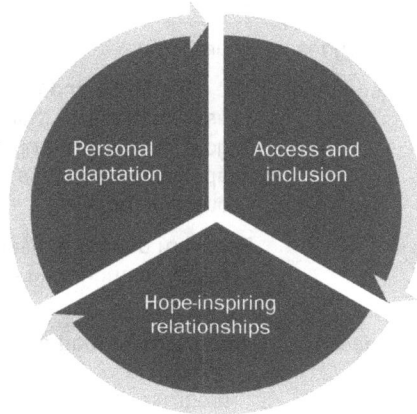

renewing work relationships and social activities, and developing new ones.
Hope-inspiring relationships involves valuing the person as they are, believing in them, and having confidence in their abilities, potential and skills. It also requires that the person is listened to and their account of experiences is believed, accepted and explored. Within hope-inspiring relationships, there is acceptance of the uncertainty of the future, and problems and setbacks are viewed as part of the process of recovery and from which we can learn and build upon (Repper and Perkins, 2003).

Repper and Perkins have also identified a range of other features within their model of recovery, which are included in Table 10.1.

Exercise

Look at the aspects of recovery outlined in Table 10.1. On a piece of paper write two headings 'Agree' and 'Disagree'. Now write down those that you agree with, and see the point of, and those you find hard to understand or that do not fit with your values (see Chapter 1).

Examples might include the notion that relapse is not a failure. Because how could a deterioration in the person's mental health be part of a positive therapeutic approach? Or that recovery is possible without professional intervention because otherwise what is the point of training as a mental health nurse? Recovery, as with all philosophies, requires thought in order to be applicable to your life and values. As we are all different, you will all have your own questions and issues with these ideas. Accept that at the end of your reflections, you may still be left with questions, not entirely convinced of the answers, or have learned something but now have a new set of questions. If so, remember them or keep a note of them and return to them in the future.

Table 10.1 Aspects of recovery according to Repper and Perkins (2003)

Feature	Description
Recovery is different for everyone	There is no recipe for success
Recovery is not about an end point	The experience and process of recovery are essential, rather than reaching a final goal. It is typified by an attitude and approach as opposed to a measurable outcome or goal
Recovery is not cure	Recovery does not mean that symptoms cease, though they may interfere less with life
Recovery is not a linear process	Improvement may not always be in uniform or consistently unbroken forward progress. There may be setbacks or reversals
Recovery is not specific to people with mental health problems	The experience of loss, bereavement, reversal and disappointment occur to most people through life. We are all recovering from life
Recovery is about taking control	Mental health problems are often seen as being typified by a loss of control. Recovery represents the process of taking back control
Recovery is about growth	There is life beyond the narrow constrictions of a mental health diagnosis. Through experiencing recovery we learn about ourselves as people
Relapse is not a failure but part of a process	The new learning we undergo as a result of experiencing crisis could not have occurred any other way. Crisis often precedes progress and an advancement in our learning
Recovery is not limited to one theory	Recovery does not involve committing to a particular theory or explanation of mental health problems. People will arrive at or value different understandings
Recovery is possible without professional intervention	The person's independent resources are significant. It is possible to recover with, without, or in spite of professional intervention

Source: Adapted from Repper and Perkins (2003).

Exercise

Think of other ways you could facilitate and include service users in their chosen environment.

- What limitations to environmental inclusion are you likely to face with your service user in terms of risks, current presentation and medications?
- How would you overcome these limitations to ensure your service user is included in their chosen environments because the inclusion is valuable and important to their recovery?

All these and many more activities can be facilitated by mental health nurses to promote the inclusion of service users within their chosen communities. This inclusion and partnership work, on the other hand, help in developing and building the therapeutic rapport necessary to enhance the nurse–patient relationship essential for the recovery of the individual. Paying close attention to service users' everyday social activities not only gives a picture of the challenges and obstacles being faced. It also demonstrates an awareness of the sociological contribution to mental health and well-being that is often overlooked or not really thought about (Davidson, 2005; Tucker, 2010).

Social inclusion is, therefore, another important principle as people do not recover in isolation (Borg and Davidson, 2008; Shepherd et al., 2008). Service users ought to be able to take on purposeful, valuable and rewarding social roles in the community. This would not only promote recovery for the individual but would access a wide-ranging and valuable pool of human experience that is often not available to the wider public. Recovery also creates the opportunity for the service user to discover or rediscover a sense of personal identity, separate from illness or disability (Borg and Davidson, 2008; Slade, 2009).

Conclusion

In this chapter we have looked at nursing models. Particular emphasis has been paid to exploring the Tidal Model and Repper and Perkins' Psychosocial Model. Although the Tidal Model is more widely practised within mental health nursing, the Psychosocial Model is recognizable as being evident in the practice of community mental health nurses, because of its recovery-based principles.

Inevitably as you move forward into qualified practice and gain in experience, your understanding and relationship to the concept of recovery will change. These same words will mean different things to you in the future than they did before. This is because you will have encountered different situations that will have made an impact on your feelings, and left an impression on you as a person. This may affect you positively or negatively. Yet this highlights something very important. Recovery synthesizes high-minded concepts of ethics and principles, with the often stark and mundane realities of biopsycho-social health. In practice settings, we are often dealing with basic problems and helping service users find the resources to meet their needs for living. Or, in other cases, trying to help service users find the desire to continue to live.

The wide and diverse role of being a mental health nurse will inevitably challenge your motivation and test you as a person. It is important to remember why you joined the profession, what it is that you continue to give, and where you find fulfilment, and to remember the maxim from the oracle at Delphi and to 'know thyself' (Chapter 4). Recovery is about being human and does not represent an antidote or cure. This can have the effect of making us feel vulnerable and unconvinced. Often theories on health are confidently couched in highly scientific terms, and aim to convince us of the power of cure and that we can eradicate disease. In the end, all we have is ourselves and that is perhaps enough.

11 The WRAP and PATH models of recovery

Adrian Thackeray

Introduction

At the heart of genuine recovery-focused care planning lies a philosophy of hope. Without a hopeful vision, it is likely that the care process will remain focused on deficit, diagnosis and maintenance. Collaboration is essential within recovery-oriented mental health if service users are to be meaningfully included in their care and to participate in a way in which they feel empowered and able to generate sustainable change and benefit (de Silva, 2011).

Mental health problems often deprive a person of hope and aspiration for the future of a life outside the mental health services. It is the role of the mental health nurse to join the person in their present suffering, without judgement or preconceptions and recognize the person's true personality. In practice, thinking about the person's hopes and dreams is often relegated behind a primary concern with risk and the management of symptoms and signs. While this is important, it ought not to be the sole focus and ambition of the service.

The aim of this chapter is to expound an understanding of practical recovery principles through the consideration of two recovery planning tools; the 'Wellness and Recovery Action Plan' (WRAP) and 'Planning Alternative Tomorrows with Hope' (PATH). An explanation is offered of the background to each of these approaches. The chapter then takes us on a step-by-step guide through these approaches. By the end of this chapter readers will:

- have developed an understanding of the philosophy of PATH and WRAP;
- appreciate how WRAP and PATH can be used in practice;
- recognize the contribution of WRAP and PATH to service users' mental well-being as valuable recovery-focused approaches in mental health nursing.

WRAP

WRAP is a sequence of action plans that emphasize wellness and improve a person's quality of life through meaningful contingency planning. WRAP was created as a result of Mary Ellen Copeland's curiosity concerning the diverse coping styles of people with mental health problems. Following being diagnosed with manic depression (now known as bipolar affective disorder), Copeland initially sent out questionnaires to service users asking how they coped and received a large response. Copeland identified core themes among the responses that later became the founding concepts of WRAP. Pleased with the responses and journey she was undertaking, Copeland explained to her psychiatrist at the time that she wished to continue and write a book on the subject, but was informed that she was being grandiose. Yet Copeland's enthusiasm was not dampened and in 1997 she was part of a group of people at a workshop in Northern Vermont, USA. The service users had come together to share ideas about wellness. Jessie Parker, one of those attending the workshop, felt that the ideas and concepts being discussed needed to be organized into a manageable format, and as a result WRAP was developed.

WRAP is a meaningful series of personal resources and action plans created by the service user. Its main focus is to provide the service user with constructive, strengths-based tools and action plans to assist in maintaining positive mental health. It also has the power to increase self-esteem and help the service user overcome varying states ranging from a dip in mood to a significant crisis. Essentially, WRAP empowers the service user when often uncertainty is never very far away. WRAP is strongly underpinned by five key concepts which are also important values that the professional working with the service user should demonstrate within the therapeutic process. These are: hope, personal responsibility, education, self-advocacy and support (Copeland, 2015).

These concepts are readily familiar to mental health nurses, as they clearly echo recovery-focused principles (Roberts and Boardman, 2014). Facilitating the WRAP approach with a service user provides them with greater opportunity to build self-agency and acknowledges the person as being an expert by experience. WRAP promotes holistic practice where every aspect of the person is involved, from the emotional to the spiritual. WRAP is often facilitated on an individual basis with the service user, or in a group. Yet consistent with our discussion in Chapter 3 about using technology, it has also emerged in different media; for example, the 'WRAP APP', which is available for smartphone users and an online version, which can be located at https://wrap.essentiallearning. cm/Default.aspx.

Making a start with WRAP

The stages of WRAP are as follows:

1 Wellness Toolbox
2 Daily Maintenance Plan
3 Triggers
4 Early Warning Signs
5 When Things Begin to Break Down
6 Crisis Plan
7 Post-Crisis Plan.

Wellness Toolbox

Essentially, WRAP contains a unique and meaningful list of activities, both of the past and of the present, which keep the person feeling well. The service user is the sole author of the *Wellness Toolbox*. It is an important starting point for the rest of the WRAP process, as it lays foundations which will support the individual through times of difficulty.

A variety of types of toolboxes are possible. Some people with creative talents may prefer to have a literal box, inside which are contained objects that symbolize wellness activities. Others may simply create a list on a piece of paper. Suggestions from friends and people who know the service user well may be included; however, ensuring the exclusivity and ownership of this work as belonging to and meaningful for the service user is essential.

EXAMPLE QUESTIONS

'In your experience, what are the things that support you staying well?'

'We're going to discuss the activities you undertake that give you a sense of real well-being, let's list some of them together.'

Some people will make use of symbolism in the construction of their Wellness Toolbox. For example, having a small piece of Lego in their toolbox might remind the person of playing Lego with their son. Others may draw pictures of the items which have positive reminders of events or activities that bring them happiness, or have a positive association.

Case Study 11.1   Rachel

Rachel is 42 years old and has bipolar affective disorder (Type 1). She receives support from her care co-ordinator based at the Community Mental Health Team and also a Support Time Recovery (STR) worker. Her care co-ordinator suggested that WRAP might assist her in maintaining positive mental health. Rachel chose the following items to include in her Wellness Toolbox:

- Photographs of a family holiday.
- A copy of her favourite novel.
- Shells from a beach she walked along with her husband.
- A small bar of chocolate.
- Her favourite music CD.
- A poem that was given to her when she was in hospital.

Each of these items is a positive reminder and represents some of her happier times. The Wellness Toolbox, however, should not be viewed merely as a collection of keepsakes but as a powerful tool which is central to the WRAP process. The amount of time spent on the Wellness Toolbox will vary from person to person, but no part of WRAP should be rushed. Adequate time needs to be allocated, with no distractions and it ought to be carried out in a quiet, restful place where there will be no interruptions. Whatever form the WRAP takes, it remains the property of the person who has authored it and the collection of wellness resources and action plans is not to be taken by the professional.

Exercise

What would you include in your Wellness Toolbox?

Now think about why you would include these items and how they might help reaffirm your sense of identity and positive mood.

Daily Maintenance Plan

Building upon the Wellness Toolbox, the Daily Maintenance Plan provides the service user with the opportunity to consolidate their current wellness resources and focus on what they need to do on a daily basis in order to help stay well. The plan will be referred to each day by the person, and as a result they may wish to make several copies so that it can be positioned in places where it is easy to see and catches the person's attention, for example, on their fridge or by their bedside table.

EXAMPLE QUESTION

'Explain to me what you are like when you are well.'

In this stage, take the time to explore past memories of when the person felt well. Wellness may be personified by, for example, a memorable social event. Or it could be as simple as listing a collection of emotions when the person knows they are experiencing positive mental health. The person may have photographs of times when they were feeling better in themselves. These could be used to trigger discussion and also be included within the Wellness Toolbox.

The second part of the Daily Maintenance Plan involves asking the person to work with you towards identifying what needs to be done every day in order to maintain the person feeling as well as possible. Explore with the person the basic activities of daily living that are needed in order for a sense of wellness to be maintained.

Case Study 11.2   Josh

Josh is 25 years old and has psychotic depression. He lives in supported housing and is seeing his Community mental health nurse at the Team office. Josh and his CPN worked towards creating a WRAP, as Josh would often neglect his self-care and basic daily living skills. Below is a list from Josh's Daily Maintenance Plan:

- I need to make sure that I wash each morning and evening.
- I need to spend time talking on the telephone with my family each day.
- I need to play on my X-box each day for at least 30 minutes.
- I need to play my guitar each day.
- Before I go to bed I need to make sure I have a wash and get changed into nightwear.

It may assist when formulating the plan to break down the day into three different sections to be able to micro-manage what the person needs to do at specific times. There may be a time of day for some people that they find particularly difficult and planning at this point may need to be more focused and specific than at other times. It can often be the most basic activities that need to be included, such as tending to personal hygiene, or keeping up with the laundry. Conversely, the person may need to write their diary every day and undertake a piece of creative work. These will be personal to the service user. It is necessary though for the mental health nurse to be prepared to learn a great deal about the person as the WRAP process unfolds. The Daily Maintenance Plan is referred to every day in the initial stages of using WRAP, and so has to be practical and useful and something that will be referred to regularly.

Exercise

Think about a time when you felt down or low in mood. Even if you have not experienced a mental health issue, sometimes we all feel down. Think back to when this was, and use this same example for the exercises in each of the stages that follow.

What would you identify in your Daily Maintenance Plan?

Triggers

Triggers cause the service user to experience an adverse, negative and distressing reaction. They come from a variety of sources including interpersonal relationships, the workplace and the local (and wider) community and can produce unanticipated effects. Supporting the service user to identify their personal triggers, and formulating an action plan for how they are going to manage these provide a helpful contingency plan to handle unexpected events. Ways to open dialogue on the subject of triggers can be as follows:

EXAMPLE QUESTIONS

'Let's turn now to less positive times – think about events in the past when something has happened that really affected you in a negative way.'

'What would you describe as your triggers? Are there any things that cause you to be seriously affected and change how you feel?'

Exploring the reaction and consequence builds a full picture of the cause and effect for the service user, and requires a strong therapeutic relationship founded on trust. The journey back to situations where the service user has experienced an adverse reaction should be treated with compassion, understanding and respect. If the process triggers emotions in the service user, the mental health nurse needs to offer support. Active listening and affirming the person's emotions and responses will show them that you empathize, are committed and present for the person, and have their best interests at heart.

Case Study 11.1   Rachel (*continued*)

Rachel found the triggers section particularly difficult but recognized that it was something she needed to go through in order to prepare for future occurrences. With support from the mental health nurse, she described the following as experiences that had made her feel upset or that were difficult for her to deal with.

Rachel identified that dealing with authority figures was a particular issue for her and caused her a great deal of anxiety and stress. She felt this was due to emotional abuse she experienced from her father when she was a child. For Rachel, speaking with the pastor at her local church caused her so much anxiety that she would actively avoid him.

Other triggers involved having to wait a long time to be served in the local post office, and at home if her mobile telephone rang and showed 'number withheld'; she would immediately presume the worst and think it was going to be bad news.

Writing all the triggers down and numbering each one assists in ordering the next step of planning actions to remedy them. The service user has the resources to find solutions to the triggers though this may require support and facilitation. The mental health nurse may offer some suggestions based on their knowledge of the service user's coping strategies, but it is essential that they do not take over. There is a wide range of different options in planning for triggers. The mental health nurse may have heard of the same trigger many times but the action plan that is chosen will reflect the individuality, uniqueness and personal preferences of the service user. Spend time with the person exploring ways they can cope with the trigger, and also consider other resources that the service user could use, including the support of family, friends and their wider social network.

Exercise

Are there any triggers in the situation that you used in the exercise above that you can identify about yourself?

If so, write these down and consider how you might cope better with these.

Early Warning Signs

Often people fail to notice the small changes, or tell-tale signs that pre-empt a deterioration in their mental health. Yet this is exactly what we do at this stage of the WRAP. The intention is to develop a contingency plan that can be used and successfully prevent this being the beginning of an inexorable decline in the service user's mental health. At first it may take time for the person to think through the signs that show a negative change in their mental health, however, as the focus on this becomes stronger, it will become easier.

EXAMPLE QUESTIONS

'Let's look now at your early warning signs – what signs do you notice that show you that things are not okay with you?'

'Are there any signs which show you that you may need to take action to avoid your mental health getting worse?'

Case Study 11.2   Josh (*continued*)

Josh was easily able to explain that he always knew when his mood was beginning to deteriorate, as he began to buy excessive amounts of takeaway meals rather than cook for himself. Not only did this demonstrate to him that his mood was lowering, but he had previously incurred debts on his credit card. Using this section of his WRAP Josh was able to make a plan of action that included ensuring that he telephoned his mother, Christine and ask her to help him by coming to his flat and preparing food with him and looking after his card during these periods.

Case Study 11.1   Rachel (*continued*)

Rachel's early warning signs of her mood becoming higher showed through her taking on more household activities than she could possibly achieve. She would then begin a cycle of derogatory and negative thinking about herself. This would drive her to an unrelenting cleaning and tidying regime that seemingly had no conclusion or satisfaction for her. Through WRAP Rachel was able to put in place measures to prevent the cycle continuing through not deviating from a list containing all the cleaning jobs she needed to undertake. Eventually she was able to plan to visit a friend when she felt the urge to clean more. She also utilized more resources from her Wellness Toolbox including writing more frequently in her Journal, and 'prayer soaking' (listening to relaxation music while praying).

Numbering the individual early warning signs along with the action plans will keep the WRAP methodical and logically sequenced, which also makes it easier to use. Early warning signs are important, and the opportunity they represent in arresting a deterioration in the service user's mental health cannot be underestimated.

Exercise

Linked to the same example identified in the previous exercise, can you think of any early warning signs of problems that you have experienced?

What were they?

What measures might help you address them?

When things begin to break down or get worse

The aim of this section is to recognize and bring clarity to the behaviours and feelings the service user has as they begin to enter the stages of crisis. Remember that one person's early warning signs may be no more than that and even if they persist, a crisis might not occur. For another person their mental health often deteriorates rapidly and dramatically following seemingly quite innocuous early signs. If the level of the distress, distraction and upset behind the sign is very high, it is likely that things are beginning to break down or get worse beyond what we are seeing. Some examples could be as follows:

- Strong compulsion towards suicide or deliberate self-harm.
- Increase in prevalence and command nature of a person's voices.
- Isolating behaviours and strongly held paranoid beliefs.

- Increasing behaviours that may jeopardize the safety of the person.
- Increasing intensity in feelings of fear and dread.
- Increased illicit drug/substance use.

While WRAP has its own crisis plan and advance directive, this section makes the assumption that the service user can still make their own decisions and they are not, at this stage, totally overcome and requiring their advance directive to be put into action.

Case Study 11.2   Josh (*continued*)

Josh found that a strong increase in a particular commanding voice instructing him to drink alcohol and self-harm was a sign that things were breaking down. 'Zach' is the most derogatory and negative towards him out of a group of four voices he experiences. Considering that he previously had serious issues with alcohol and dangerous behaviours associated with this, the emergence of a specific voice encouraging him to harm himself with a Stanley knife was not to be ignored. When the voice had previously instructed him, he had been unable to resist the temptation to drink and would become intoxicated leading to an increased likelihood of his carrying out self-harm. Josh and his mental health nurse were able to implement a plan should he experience 'Zach'. First, he agreed to contact the crisis team and explain the situation. Second, he would telephone his mother who would drive to Josh's flat and provide him with some respite at her home. Josh decided he would watch television when at his mother's, as it made him feel relaxed. He also decided that he would undertake artwork as it helps to distract him from his voices.

The Wellness Toolbox is essential as a repertoire of useful coping strategies cannot be overemphasized at this stage in the planning process. It can be drawn upon again and again to provide positive coping mechanisms and also serve as a pool of resources to draw upon when things break down. For this reason the service user may wish to keep copies of the list of resources in prominent places.

Exercise

In relation to the same situation used in the previous exercises, in hindsight, what would you say made things go from bad to worse?

Now think about what you might have been able to do in that situation.

Personal Crisis Plan

Advance directives in mental healthcare have become a subject of significant debate (Jankovic et al., 2010). This section of WRAP allows the wishes and preferences of the service user to be clear and unambiguous.

Working collaboratively on the crisis plan will take a significant amount of time, and it is essential that the work is not influenced by the mental health nurse but remains the sole work of the service user. Again time needs to be allocated to complete it in a suitably peaceful, private and undisturbed environment while the final Crisis Plan needs to be distributed to those who may need to be involved.

Part One   What I am like when I am well?

This description will have already been made at other stages of the WRAP and so these details can be taken from the earlier work.

Part Two   Indicators that I need assistance from others

In this part of the WRAP, actions considered to increase the risk of harm to the service user or others are described. These include illicit substance misuse, grandiose beliefs, impetuosity, and risky or self-harming behaviours. Referring to the 'when things are breaking down' section may assist in developing this part of the WRAP.

Part Three   Supporters

The person's supporters are essential to the success of the Crisis Plan. It is necessary to discuss reasons for the inclusion of certain people; however, the professional must not coerce the service user into making a particular selection. A minimum of five people is advantageous, and speaking to them will help to clarify and agree the expectations, commitment and any particular instructions or requirements that the service user might have. The person's name, relationship to the service user and details of their specific role should be clearly documented.

Part Four   Medication

Invite the person you are working with to list all the medications they take together with times, dosages and reasons why they take them. In addition, note which medications they are willing to take in crisis situations, and those that they do not wish to be prescribed under any circumstances – it is within this section that allergies and sensitivities can be documented.

Part Five   Treatments

Considering the vast array of potential treatment options, ask the service user to list all treatments that they will accept as appropriate for them, and clearly state those which they resolutely do not wish to have.

Part Six   Home, Community and Respite

WRAP supports community-based care wherever possible (Copeland, 2014). This makes sense as recovery is easier if the person has never been away from their familiar surroundings to begin with, therefore this stage of the WRAP specifically focuses on community-based care. Ask the service user to speak with their supporters, to ascertain how much time they could spend with the service user if they needed more intensive help. Or if the service user wishes to spend time with relatives, this too could be discussed with them.

Part Seven   Treatment Facilities

In some cases hospitalization is needed, although this should not be the first option. Where this is the case, preferred treatment facilities can be listed. This allows the service user to still have some control in circumstances where this is often not the case. It is important to discuss who they would want to be notified of their admission, arrangements for care of their pets to be considered and who they would like to assist them home upon discharge.

Part Eight   What Helps and What Doesn't

It is important to detail exactly what the service user wants from their supporters. Ask the service user to look back at their Wellness Toolbox and identify the things that help them feel well, for example, talking with a friend about a positive event, or having a special meal made for them. The more exact these details, the greater the beneficial effect the supporter will have when carrying out the service user's wishes. Conversely, being specific over what does not work and actually increases agitation is also imperative.

Part Nine   Recognizing Recovery

Highlighting signs and behaviours that inform the service user's supporters of a positive change in their well-being will identify when recovery is beginning to take place. Being explicit about these indicators, and explaining them in detail will show those involved when the crisis plan is no longer needed.

The WRAP is a detailed tool that has the potential to most importantly empower but also provide reassurance for the service user during the distressing and fearful times of relapse and crisis. Yet at the same time it is a positive tool, offering the potential to support mental well-being and engagement in activities that can keep the person well. Spending time over the WRAP will help to support the person develop self-knowledge and feel more in control of their mental health but at the same time create a valuable therapeutic resource that has multiple uses. Next we explain and discuss PATH which is another useful recovery-focused approach for working with service users.

PATH

PATH offers a method of working with service-users that focuses on their dreams, desires and ideas for a positive future. PATH first emerged in the early 1990s and was created by Jack Pearpoint, John O'Brien and Marsha Forest, who were teachers championing inclusive practice for students, regardless of individual ability (Falvey et al., 2000).

PATH offers a blank canvas of ideas and possibilities, and is person-centred planning tool. The power of hope, collaboration and the focus on the service user achieving their self-directed goals is central to the PATH philosophy. It is an individually directed planning tool based on hope, collaboration, the gift of time, and placing autonomy for decision making in the hands of the service user. Not only does it foster hope, but also with this new found optimism and confidence provides an opportunity for the service user to go further and develop their own curiosity.

For PATH to function effectively, a therapeutic connectedness between both parties is essential. A central tenet is the person achieving their own, self-directed goals through a creative map of possibilities. Facilitators of PATH will need to have completed their own PATH. Consequently, it is a tool that reinforces mutual understanding, promotes equality between the mental health nurse and service user and provides the mental health nurse with the opportunity to understand the client on a deeper level.

Making a start with PATH

The stages of PATH are as follows:

1 The Dream Map
2 The Now
3 Realistic Goals
4 Enrol
5 Nightmares
6 Strong
7 First Steps
8 Future Steps

PATH's sophistication lies in its simplicity. To begin with, all that is required is a large sheet of paper and a selection of colourful pens, a private space where there will be no interruptions, and perhaps some music of the service user's choice to generate a relaxed, informal atmosphere. If a large sheet of paper is not available, it is possible to use some A4 paper. It is helpful to explain the PATH process, for the service user to agree it might be useful and for them to wish to take part.

Part One   The Dream Map

The first sheet of paper will be used to delve into the person's inner dreams and desires for their life. This may require a variety of initial questions to assist the client into dream-based thinking.

EXAMPLE QUESTIONS

'*What sort of things did you want to do in your life before you experienced the issues that brought you here?*'

'*Imagine for a moment that you do not have the issues that brought you here, what would you be doing with your life?*'

Case Study 11.3   Louise

Louise is 18 and has generalized anxiety and attachment disorder with a developmental delay. Her PATH began while she was an inpatient on an acute mental health unit and was continued by the home treatment team. A large sheet of paper was used, and Louise was asked what her dreams were. She chose not to draw pictures or write, because she found this very difficult, but did choose the colour of the pens that were used. Louise was able to verbalize that she wanted to go to Spain, live in a hotel, be a teacher, play guitar, go swimming and be more relaxed. These dreams were drawn in words and pictures by the mental health nurse.

It is essential that whatever the person states as a dream is taken seriously and drawn on their dream map. In terms of ownership, it is preferable if the person draws their dream; however, sometimes the mental health nurse may carry this out.

The mental health nurse should maintain a genuine curiosity in each dream idea that is expressed by the service user. Positive affirmation and interest in the service user's dream ideas demonstrate a wish to enter the service user's world. It helps to explore each dream in order to maintain the sense of possibility. Often the service user may become more animated and enthusiastic as they give themselves permission to explore their deepest wishes and life desires and these gain a sense of possibility.

The mental health nurse needs to remain aware of their own reactions to what the service user shares. These represent the person's most treasured dreams, thoughts and wishes and offence may easily be taken, even to comments or responses that are not intended disrespectfully.

Part Two   The Now

The session now shifts from the imagined future to the realism of the present moment. Asking the person to describe their 'now' represents a marked departure, which needs to be clearly pointed out by the mental health nurse. Some people enjoy the opportunity to discuss their current situation. Yet others prefer to keep discussion of the 'now' as simple demographics – how old they are, where they live and diagnosis. It is important to respect the service user's choice and to accept this at face value, as opposed to questioning further and pushing for more.

'We're going to make a major turn now, I'd like you to leave the dreams and your future and come back to the present – how would you describe your life now?'

'Coming back to the present moment – we're going to look at your life and how it is for you right now. Can you tell me a bit about your life and how things are for you in the present?'

Eleanor Longden is an ex-service user who now works as a clinical psychologist in Bradford and is active in promoting recovery-based practice. She describes how a breakthrough in her recovery came from a professional gently correcting her when she began to describe herself in terms that others had used. The professional asked her who *she* said she was, not what *others* said she was (Longden, 2011). Identifying subtle, yet significant nuances in the service user's thinking that have an impact on their self-perception may provide the potential for therapeutic progress. In the same way the mental health nurse needs to continually reflect, and be aware of what they are learning and gaining in knowledge through working with the service user (see Chapter 4).

> **Case Study 11.3   Louise (*continued*)**
>
> Louise chose to put on her 'now' that she was currently in hospital, aged eighteen and single. She also added that she mainly felt sad and that she had recently suffered the bereavement of her Nan.

The now can be drawn or put in simple words that the person chooses. Asking them to choose different colours for the different sections also provides a unique and personalized document.

Part Three   Realistic Goals

There are many things we would like to do, and if asked we could all produce a long list. Yet if we narrow this down to what we can do based on our current resources, we could still identify something worthwhile. This is the case no matter how meagre our finances or opportunities. There are still opportunities and changes we could make that we would enjoy. Furthermore, this might be something that unless asked we would never have thought of otherwise.

What will become evident through persistence in asking the person 'what else would you like to do with your life?' is a narrowing down of the bigger picture into small, meaningful possibilities the person wishes to explore. In Louise's case, her main dream was to go to Spain and live in a hotel. However, upon closer inspection, she wanted to go swimming and feel more relaxed.

EXAMPLE QUESTIONS

'Let's consider all of the dreams out on the map now, which one of these would you say you could work on at the moment?'

'You've got some amazing dreams here, but if we were to narrow this down to one or two goals that we'd look at working together on, which ones would it be?'

Case Study 11.4   Geoff

Geoff is 55 years old and has paranoid schizophrenia. He has been involved with the mental health services for the majority of his life and does not remember a time previously to living in an inpatient environment. Nursing staff had mixed feelings regarding whether PATH would assist Geoff. Some felt that discussing his dreams would not be fair on him, as it might raise his expectations, and lead to him being disappointed when these were not met. When asked, Geoff stated that he would like to own a bungalow on a plot of land that had been left to him. He went on to speak of having a girlfriend and a dog. He also described how he would work as either a policeman or own a car valeting business, and suggested he might like to go to the beach to walk his dog and would have a camper van. His dream hobbies included playing football, and he expressed a desire to learn to play the guitar.

People accessing services have a very good understanding of what they feel ready to achieve and this decision is often one of the quickest within the PATH process. For Geoff, the most realistic goal he chose was to begin to learn how to play the guitar, which he is now doing.

Part Four   Enrol

Enrolling is the point where the service user decides who they want to be a part of the desired realistic goal. This section of PATH provides a great sense of ownership, choice and collaboration. The service user, possibly for the first time in their experience of mental health services, is allowed to choose a supporter who they believe can assist them on their journey. It is beneficial to acknowledge the wider support circle as well, for example, professionals, family and friends. Being able to exercise such a degree of choice increases the likelihood of the goal being successful, as the service user is acknowledging those people with whom they have developed strong therapeutic relationships.

'Who would you choose to support you on this journey?'

'If you could choose anyone to enrol on this goal – who would it be?'

Part Five   Nightmares

Nightmares were added to the PATH by Ron Coleman and Karen Taylor, recovery consultants and campaigners based in Scotland. Exploring the worst case scenario allows the focus person to take a good look at themselves and express their fears. Louise's nightmare was that her anxiety would be so bad when she went swimming that she would not manage to even get to the pool. Louise accepted additional support from the team that helped in planning for the event. There is a strong element of contingency planning within the Nightmares section and if the service user's concerns are listened to and acted upon it, increases the likelihood of the goal being successful. For Geoff, the nightmare scenario was the prospect of experiencing electroconvulsive therapy (ECT).

EXAMPLE QUESTIONS

'What is the worst thing that could happen to prevent you realizing your goal?'

'Is there anything that could happen between now and your goal being realized that would completely upset our planned journey?'

'I respect that this may be a difficult question to answer, but can you describe your worst nightmare – particularly if we consider your goal, what could go wrong?'

Part Six   Strong

Consistent with the notion that discovering what fuels a person's sense of well-being is at the heart of the recovery process (Devonshire Partnership Trust, 2014), it is the strong section which offers a discussion that can be both surprising and highly informative. Ask the service user to describe what keeps them strong – this can be anything from a pet to a soft toy, a person or a possession that holds a memory. All of the answers can be drawn or written on a separate sheet of paper. If the service user does not have any close relationships, it may be that music, television or religious faith gives the person a sense of belonging. The purpose of this activity is to collect an array of positive options that can be a useful defence against nightmare scenarios.

Case Study 11.4   Geoff (*continued*)

Geoff surprised the mental health nurse by explaining that watching the soap opera *EastEnders* kept him feeling strong, as it reminded him of his London-based family. Listening to Pink Floyd, reading letters from friends and looking through his coin collection also gave him a positive sense of well-being.

Case Study 11.3   Louise (*continued*)

Louise explained that social media and using her smartphone were enormously important in her life. Working on a scrapbook of photographs of her nieces and nephews, card making and telephone calls were also important in helping her feel well.

The strong aspect of PATH is a powerful encounter, and identifies the tools that help the service user build themselves up, and maintain a sense of well-being. Maintaining a positive, non-judgemental stance towards this activity is essential – the only exception to this rule is if the client discloses behaviours that would harm themselves or others.

Part Seven   First Steps

The first steps stage is taking the initial actions in reaching towards the desired goal. These small steps are the activities that need to take place in the next 72 hours to make the goal become a reality. The first steps can be numbered and given special prominence through colour and larger lettering.

EXAMPLE QUESTIONS

'What are the things we need to do in the next seventy-two hours to kick-start this goal?'

'Are there any basic things we need to look into to get closer to this goal becoming a reality?'

Case Study 11.3   Louise (*continued*)

Louise wanted to go swimming. In order to make the first steps, she identified that she would need to try on her swimming costume to see if it still fits, check where the leisure centre was, how much entry into the pool would cost, and what times the female-only pool sessions were. She said she could obtain this information online.

'First steps' provide a time-directed challenge and should address practical realities.

Part Eight   Future Steps

Future steps will list the actions required to successfully complete the goal. The duration of time between the PATH being created and completion of the goal is variable. However, it is important to establish a time frame. A two- to three-week period would allow sufficient time for preparations to be made, activities to be completed and also provide time for any problems to be overcome.

EXAMPLE QUESTIONS

'What things will you need to do a week before your goal is due to be realized?'

'What are the last steps you'll need to take on this journey – are there any things you need to do after your first steps to ensure that what we've planned will take place?'

Case Study 11.3   Louise (*continued*)

For Louise to go swimming she needed to purchase a new bathing costume, and save money from her benefits to be able to afford to attend the local leisure centre. Another of her future steps was to maintain regular contact with her friend Elaine who she could talk to about her anxieties over swimming in public. This future step was established because one of Louise's nightmares was that she would not be able to enter the leisure centre, and therefore needed to acknowledge and discuss this option with someone she could rely upon and trust.

Future steps can include additional support, with specific expectations, and details of the support required. It allows the goal to stay on track and supports the service user through to completion of their goal.

Conclusion

In this chapter we have discussed WRAP and PATH, as two of the most recovery-focused therapeutic approaches. Through focusing on the positive and possible, WRAP builds a database of unique and personal recovery-focused information. If utilized sensitively and constructively, WRAP is a powerful change agent which ensures that the service user leads every step of the journey. Eliciting and recording the specific details of the plan may be time-consuming. However, the long-term benefit of crises being averted sooner than otherwise might be the case, and the service user feeling empowered when experiencing relapse cannot be overemphasized.

In contrast, PATH serves to bridge the distance between the service user's dreams and reality, and helps with life planning. Inevitably, this will benefit the service user's quality of life and also promotes feelings of empowerment, confidence, motivation, purpose and sense of self-agency. PATH provides a useful service user and recovery-focused framework with which mental health nurses can work to achieve therapeutic progress within the always present confines of limited resources.

12 The politics of recovery

Nick Wrycraft

Introduction

In this chapter we discuss the influence of politics in mental health nursing, and a recovery-focused perspective. In the past it was possible for mental health nurses to solely focus on the care of service users. Yet over the past 20 years nursing activity has become more concerned with budgets and targets and a politically driven agenda. Although intruding more than ever before into our work, politics has always been highly relevant to nursing and mental health. In spite of being numerically the largest represented profession in the health service, nursing has traditionally lacked a political profile. At the same time, many mental health nurses and students also believe that politics is not relevant to them. In this chapter we discuss how politics is relevant to mental health nursing and inextricably linked to practice and recovery.

Politics involves confronting tough choices, and these have been intensified with the increasingly straitened resources available to mental health services in recent years. While mental health is an umbrella term, some people with unpopular diagnoses, such as personality disorder and substance misuse (see Chapter 1), have experienced a lack of service provision in relation to other areas. As we discuss, the current philosophy of service design leads to a fragmented system that is inconsistent.

In the chapter we look at some of the history of the mental health services within the National Health Service (NHS). This demonstrates that mental health provision is profoundly political, yet too often overlooked. Often changes have occurred reactively, and in response to significant unmet need or public concern. For mental health services to be more effective, a more proactive approach is required. A cohesive and overarching plan is required to create services of the future, as opposed to continually striving to meet outstanding needs of the present. The first step towards achieving this is for mental health to be more of a priority. Mental health nurses can contribute towards this by embodying recovery-based values in everything that they do, and placing service users at the centre of their care.

By the end of this chapter we will have discussed:

- what politics means, and how you as an individual engage with it;
- the complex relationship between the government, mental health services and people with mental health issues;

- the ways in which politics is evident in everyday practice, and how we might work within the limitations that this implies in a recovery-focused manner.

Politics and government

Politics is derived from the Greek word *polis*, and refers to the state and the government and the running and administration of its interests. These include the legal and justice system, education and healthcare. The government of a state reflects its values, principles and priorities. Within this, mental healthcare is a central issue.

Over recent years there has been a sense of disengagement with politics in the UK (Elledge, 2014). With the growth of technology in mass communication and increased public access to information, it might be expected that interest in politics would have increased. However, it seems that politicians are more the subject of derision and suspicion than ever (Jowitt, 2012). Among the reasons for this is that the ease and widespread availability of information can lead to confusion over what to believe, while at the same time politics has been slow to use the internet and media in a manner that presents their arguments effectively.

Q: Do you have an interest in politics?

A: If you answered 'no' to the above question, then you are by no means alone. A poll of people taken in any setting outside of a meeting of members of a political party asking whether they are interested in politics would be likely to receive a lukewarm response at best. Many people seem to be disillusioned with politics: the average turnout for a general election in the UK has declined significantly since the Second World War, and is around 60–70 per cent of everyone eligible to vote (UK Political Info, 2016). Among the reasons are the following:

- Feeling uninspired by politicians.
- A sense of apathy, and that nothing will change anyway, so why bother?
- Resentment that politicians do not represent the population from whom they are elected.
- Feeling that politicians are 'out of touch'.

Mental health is inextricably linked to politics. People with mental health issues sometimes struggle to access primary healthcare for their physical health. They are also among the groups within society most likely to experience social exclusion, be unemployed and in receipt of benefits. All of these are highly political issues, and the subject of much debate.

In addition to this, as we saw in Chapter 4, people with mental health issues are subject to the complex issue of preconception and stigma. This has potentially significant political implications. For example, some people feel that service users with substance abuse are responsible for their own situation. They may argue for criminal convictions, and punishment, and the stopping of benefits to act as a disincentive and promote behavioural change. In contrast, others believe that addiction is an illness, and cannot simply be stopped and instead advocate treatment, rehabilitation and community-based interventions as part of a comprehensive multifaceted package. Holders of both these viewpoints are also often vehemently critical of each other, and convinced that the other is wrong. Other factors such as media agendas also contribute to this situation. For example, through broadcasting stories portraying people who misuse substances in a certain light, whether it be good or bad, the media further influences public opinion. Often stigma and misconceptions develop and are propagated where certain groups are easy to identify, and those who are disapproving do not know or have direct contact with those individuals. It is hoped that politicians and those responsible for policy make decisions based on the best evidence, and the views of service users, stakeholders and professionals, as opposed to beliefs based on appeasing discrimination and misconception.

Within healthcare generally, there is immense overall need, yet only finite resources. When seeking to raise awareness of mental health, it is not simply enough to believe that this will be a self-evident priority for politicians. If we do not take part, we never have the opportunity to make a change. Also, as we discussed in Chapter 2, it is necessary to always have hope as a fundamental attribute of recovery. While it is wise to recognize when a task is beyond our capabilities, it does not automatically follow that because something looks unlikely to change that we should just give up. Hope provides a glimpse of the possible, establishes a basis for optimism, and sense of opportunity that things might change. Being politically active also allows us to express ourselves. As we discussed in Chapter 3, an important aspect of communication is simply sharing with others, so that while we might not find a ready-made answer to problems, knowing that another person shares the same feelings and views helps. Politicians, however, often present facts and statistics to back their arguments; these are normally selected because they support the policy or proposal they favour. While this depends on the particular issue that is being discussed, the future has yet to happen. So no matter how confident or certain politicians seem to be, we can never be sure that their preferred course of action is the correct one.

Often political legacies are determined by unexpected events; for example, the Brexit vote (Foster, 2017), therefore in spite of the assured appearances and confidence of politicians, it could be said that politics is as much about instinct, feeling, emotion and ultimately timing as well-thought out plans, facts and statistics. Choosing not to be involved in politics only compounds feelings of powerlessness and resentment. This can lead the gaps and inequalities in socio-economic prosperity and health to widen, and for people to continue to feel disgruntled because they feel that society does not represent their viewpoint (Marmot Review, 2010).

In this section of the chapter, we have considered what politics is, and looked at why many people are feeling apathetic and powerless, but also begun to discuss why it makes sense to take part and be involved. If we are to practise from a recovery-based perspective, we need to fully embrace this philosophy personally. Doing so involves looking at how hopeful we feel, and communicating this as a means to provide reassurance and foster social cohesion. Engaging in politics is important; some would even say it is an obligation. If we are to increase public participation and awareness, then we as professionals need to take an active role and present a good example. Participation can take different forms but begins by becoming informed through listening, reading and keeping up with the news. It might also include:

- becoming aware of what the political parties stand for and reading their manifestos;
- voting;
- discussing politics and political issues with friends, family and peers;
- maybe even joining a political party, attending meetings and getting involved in events.

In the next part of the discussion, we consider the development of the NHS and the mental health services.

The NHS

People have always needed the same basic resources in order to live and function healthily. These ensure our continued existence and prosperity. The essentials for health at its most basic level include safety and security, physical health and well-being, and environmental resources, for example, decent and affordable housing and amenities, but also affordable food and sustenance and a clean water supply. All of these appear on the lower levels of Maslow's (1943) hierarchy (see Figure 12.1). Often we take these basic resources for granted. Sanitation and a clean water supply have not always existed, and in some parts of the world today still do not exist, creating a challenge for people simply to remain alive. However, sometimes there are deficits even in the most basic of areas. For example, currently there is a shortage of suitable and affordable housing for many younger people in the UK. Large inequalities in health continue to exist between different regions of the UK. The Marmot Review (2010) reiterated the long-established trend of people in poorer areas of the UK experiencing higher levels of deprivation being prone to worse mental and physical health outcomes. Health status and social needs on the one hand, and personal and economic resources on the other, are important factors in determining the nature of health issues. Sadly, for many there is a constant battle to meet and provide for their everyday needs, often while experiencing physical and/or mental health issues. Many others enjoy a good standard of living and level of comfort that satisfies their needs.

Figure 12.1 Maslow's hierarchy of need

Source: https://upload.wikimedia.org/wikipedia/commons/thumb/6/60/Maslow%27s_Hierarchy_ of_Needs.svg/1280px-Maslow%27s_Hierarchy_of_Needs.svg.png.

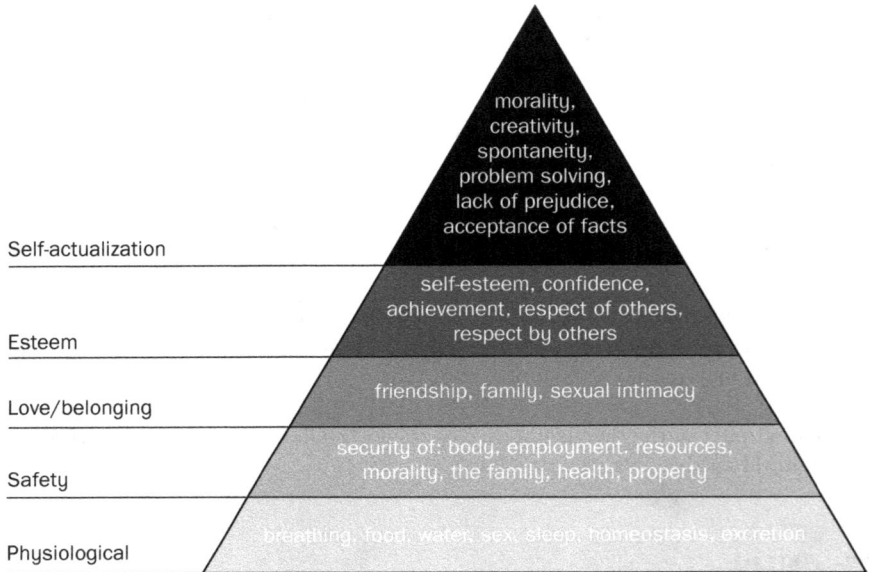

Exercise

Look at the hierarchy in Figure 12.1. Where would you place yourself on Maslow's hierarchy of needs?

For most people the single most important political initiative in healthcare in the UK in the twentieth century was the creation of the NHS in 1948. Following the Second World War, and as a result of the Beveridge Report of 1942, the then Health Secretary Aneurin Bevin introduced the NHS. The principle on which it was based was that treatment was free to all at the point of access. This was a groundbreaking initiative as it demonstrated a commitment on the part of the state to the health of its individuals. This is a fundamental, yet crucial principle that many still regard as extremely important and valuable.

The NHS was introduced for numerous good reasons. These included:

- a generally shared sense that the existing mixed system of part private and part public-funded healthcare was not working;
- as a result of the Second World War the health services had become better developed and more responsive, and a national health service seemed to be logical;

- a sense of optimism and desire in the post-war period to develop good basic services for the whole population;
- a desire to provide a uniform and nationwide healthcare system to allow basic standards of healthcare support.

However, when introduced, it was envisaged that most major health problems and diseases would be eradicated within 10 years, and as opposed to a service dedicated to illness, the NHS would eventually be focused on health promotion. Due to the sheer scope and range of services the NHS provided, and the continuing burden of ill-health, the consequences of the commitment involved were greater than anyone could have initially anticipated. From the outset, there were significant costs in supporting the service, and these steadily escalated over time. Eventually, associated services, which were originally provided for free by the NHS, such as dentistry, eye tests, and even regular prescriptions, were paid for by the patient. Over recent decades the costs of healthcare have continued to rise, and there have also been advances in technology. Additionally, the internet has led to patients becoming more informed, aware of choices of treatments, and having higher and more expensive expectations of healthcare and the NHS. The combination of these factors has led some to question the sustainability of the NHS in the future.

Consequently, there is a persistent fear among supporters of the NHS of the abandonment of the principle of treatment free for all at the point of access and the introduction of privatization of services. These emotive and important arguments have often hampered the wide-ranging and creative thinking necessary to develop and run an effective health service in the twenty-first century. This has not been helped, however, by the highly political orientation of the reforms of the 1980s onwards and the introduction of the internal free market that has led to frequent murmurs of concern at privatization 'by the back door'. In the next part of this chapter we look more specifically at mental health within the NHS.

The NHS and mental health

In 1948 the mental health services were included within health for the first time, having previously been under the remit of social care. During the 1950s the inpatient population was also peaking with more than 150,000 mental health inpatient beds in the UK (Jones, 1993). Due to the sheer number of inpatient admissions and cost of maintaining and caring for this number of people, change was clearly necessary. Yet it came as a surprise when in 1962 the then Secretary of State for Health Enoch Powell announced the closure of the asylums, and over the next four decades community care was developed (Jones, 1993). However, internationally, there was an overall move away from an institutional model of care to a more community-based approach.

The reason for this sudden and massive change in government policy was propelled by a number of factors:

- Most compelling of all was the sheer cost, not only of supporting the large number of inmates within institutions and lack of turnaround through people not being discharged, but the upkeep and maintenance of large and deteriorating buildings.
- Social attitudes became more liberal and public opinion nationally and internationally recognized that institutional care was outdated. In the early 1960s several books were published by influential writers in different countries, all of whom were highly critical of mental health institutions. These included Michel Foucault's (1989) *Madness and Civilization*, R. D. Laing's (1970) *The Divided Self*, Thomas Szasz's (1961) *Myth of Mental Illness* and Erving Goffman's (1960) *Asylums*.
- The development of effective medication and psychological therapies meant that people experiencing long-term mental health problems could be supported in the community, instead of requiring a hospital environment.

(Adapted from Jones, 1993)

Yet it was not until the 1980s and 1990s that institutions began to close down, and the development of care in the community gathered momentum. Some argued strongly that the government saw this policy just as a means of saving money, as opposed to representing a preferable and well-planned alternative to institutional care. A number of high-profile tragic incidents, such as Benjamin Silcock, who was severely injured after climbing into the lion enclosure at London Zoo, and Jonathan Zito, who was killed by Christopher Clunis, a mental health service user, revealed major flaws in the service.

Sustained public pressure eventually led to government action, with the introduction of the Care Programme Approach (CPA) in 1990 (see below). This was an attempt to provide an integrated network for mental health services that were accountable, inclusive and provided some sense of multidisciplinary and multi-agency integration. At the same time the computerization of health records meant that CPA could be more effectively implemented and monitored. CPA remains an influential feature of the mental health services today, and, while having advantages and disadvantages, is useful for setting standards and providing a framework for mental healthcare.

We have already reflected upon the first two levels of Maslow's (1943) *Hierarchy of Needs* (see Figure 12.1), and thought about where we might be placed. In order to ascend to the higher levels, though, people need to experience, for example, love and belonging, self-esteem and self-actualization at the apex of the pyramid. It is likely that there is a high level of direct intervention regarding physical resources in the lower levels of Maslow's hierarchy. For example, we all need water, food, shelter and housing. Yet the higher levels involve more individualized psychosocial interventions.

Most of us would feel that a rewarding life is composed of much more than the basic resources that we need to live and support ourselves, and meeting the requirements of the first two levels of Maslow's pyramid.

Exercise

Look at levels 3 and 4 of Maslow's hierarchy of needs, in Figure 12.1.

- *Level 4*: Esteem: self-esteem, confidence, achievement, respect of others, respect by others.
- *Level 3*: Love/belonging: friendship, family, sexual intimacy.

1 Which of these aspects are important to you and why?
2 Which of these aspects are present in your life?
3 Which of these aspects would you like to be more evident in your life?
4 How can you go about developing these aspects to a greater extent?

When considering the higher levels, we are all different in terms of our needs and preferences for friendship, love, feeling valued by others and how we engage with society. People with mental health issues often experience difficulties forming and maintaining relationships. This may be a result of symptoms. For example, anxiety and paranoia can cause problems for the person feeling comfortable establishing a rapport, trusting or even being with others. Or the person may have experienced social stigma and exclusion that lead to longer-term feelings of rejection and fear and a reluctance to re-engage with society. They may also feel ashamed and embarrassed and choose to remove themselves from contact with others as a result. Though it is also the case, and this can apply to those with or without a mental health issue, that some people simply do not want to engage with others in social relationships, but instead prefer to lead a solitary existence.

Yet it is also the case that people often live in the community in very difficult and lonely situations, and may be experiencing paranoia or delusions that leads them to be reluctant to engage with others. If I continue to meet my self-care and physical health needs, secondary mental health services may not become involved. This is not to suggest that the scope of the law ought to be expanded to make social inclusion compulsory. Although it might seem obvious, it is hard to differentiate between what our basic needs are, and those that we need to satisfy in order to continue to live, and those we need to satisfy in order to lead a good quality of life and feel fulfilled. A consequence of this is that perhaps we need to reflect on our notion of social inclusion, and what this means and how we can apply it to our work with service users.

In the next part of the chapter we look at the development of mental health services in the NHS and the National Service Framework for Mental Health.

The National Service Framework for Mental Health

In the late 1990s the government announced a series of National Service Frameworks (NSFs) for various areas of healthcare. The second of these was for mental health, and for the first time a clear set of national standards was established providing expectations of services and the level of care that might be expected of the mental health services. *The National Service Framework for Mental Health* (DoH, 1999) prioritized timely assessment for those with ongoing mental health needs, and the provision of appropriate care planning and regular evaluations and reviews of care. Furthermore, the role of mental health services in the promotion of mental health, and assessing and planning for the needs of carers and their significant others represented a major step forward in the recognition of the scope of the role of the mental health services. The CPA represents a useful means by which the priorities of the NSF could be carried out. CPA requires that all users of specialist secondary mental health services are assessed, that their care is planned on the basis of this assessment, and that a named care co-ordinator offers a consistent point of contact. Regular evaluations of the care plan are also carried out, and the needs of carers are assessed as a part of the package (NHS Choices, undated). Disappointingly, anecdotal experience suggests that in practice the assessment of the needs of carers and significant others is often not meaningfully carried out. Mental health promotion, however, has always sat outside the remit of secondary mental health.

The failure to fully implement the aspirations of the *National Service Framework for Mental Health* (DoH, 1999) perhaps illustrates the widely held perception of a lack of commitment of successive governments to mental health. Over the years since the NSF was introduced, secondary mental health services have become progressively more one-dimensional and overspecialized, while physical healthcare dominates the priorities and distribution of funding within the NHS. Mental health constitutes 28 per cent of the disease burden incumbent on the nation yet receives only 13 per cent of the health budget (Triggle, 2014). The lack of parity between mental and physical healthcare has been a recurrent and ongoing issue, and repeatedly conceded as a problem by the government (NHS, 2014). The implication of this in practice is that three-quarters of people with a mental health issue receive little or no treatment, while people with mental health issues have a lower life expectancy of between 15–20 years compared to others (King's Fund, 2016).

There has been a wide range of government action in order to address the lack of parity between physical and mental health:

- The government passed the Health and Social Care Act (UK Government, 2012) to promote equal focus on mental health by 2020.
- The 'No Health Without Mental Health' strategy (HM Government, 2011).
- In April 2015, waiting times have been introduced in mental health for the first time with waiting times being measured for the Improving Access to Psychological Therapies (IAPT) and Early Intervention in Psychosis (EiP) services (King's Fund, 2016).
- There has been an emphasis on improving crisis services in response to a shortage of beds, variations in response across regions and in police services (DoH, 2014).

- This trend has been continued with the announcement of the new five-year plan by the Independent Mental Health Task Force to the NHS in England in February, 2016 (NHS England, 2016).

While the above interventions represent positive action, often in the documents the picture of mental health services makes daunting reading. This could be seen as an attempt to temper expectations but also suggests that there is doubt even among the policy-makers that the service will be significantly improved.

In the mental health policy pronouncements of successive governments since 1999, there has been a disappointing move away from a unified and integrated approach. In order to address the marginalized and poor relative status of mental health, what is required is greater government commitment for the rhetoric to become a reality (King's Fund, 2016). In clinical practice there is very limited cross-agency working, due to the highly specialist remits of these teams. Without an overarching and integrated vision of mental health services, provision exists as a loose affiliation of specialist services. Service users, such as those with dual diagnosis, co-morbid substance misuse or needs that do not fit neatly into specialist categories risk being passed from service to service, or worse, finding that there is no service at all for their need. At the same time, people with intermittent needs, who in the past may have received ongoing support from community mental health nurses, are often discharged completely from care once the crisis has resolved. This means that in the event of future crises, they have to go through the whole process of being re-referred and reassessed, leading to time being wasted and people remaining in avoidable distress.

From our discussion so far, it is evident that politics has the potential to exert a significant impact on the design and structure of mental health services, through making ideas a reality. This can have both positive and negative impacts. Certainly services for mental health are very much shaped with a clear notion of the target group that these resources serve. A consequence though of more recent policy is that some groups of service users have their needs overlooked and not provided for. *The National Service Framework for Mental Health* (DoH, 1999) saw mental health as a cohesive whole. It could be argued that we now have a more specialized service based on a philosophy of individuated care pathways. However, an ideological inconsistency is that in order to do this on a national service level, standardized pathways need to be developed that lose focus on the individual. This contradicts a philosophy of recovery, and places the needs of the service above those of the user. A further consequence is that there is a fragmented service.

What is needed is a more developed view of mental health services, which sees the service as a totality, and which promotes coherent links between tiers of the service. Sadly, the history of the mental health services within the NHS as we have traced it so far in this chapter is dominated by political concerns. It has largely been characterized by a risk-averse approach that reacts to public opinion and is dominated by preoccupations about cost and short-term performance indicators. These concerns and criteria are not consistent with a recovery approach, or the long-term development of a sustainable service. Often mental health service users are involved with multiple agencies and measuring the service user's progress can be complex.

Mental health policy needs to demonstrate connections between mental health problems and mental health promotion and well-being. The striking rates of relapse of most mental health issues suggests a lack of relapse prevention planning, which will be remedied by not only supporting service users through their crisis but beyond, and setting in place long-term plans for recovery. At the heart of the apparent caution of mental health policy seems to be a concern that if we open the floodgates, there will be a catastrophic torrent of demand for mental health services. There is, however, another way of looking at this issue, for example, to develop a comprehensive and integrated service focused on the individuals who need it. Not only will we reduce their distress and that of their families, carers and significant others but we will benefit society and perhaps ease overburdened secondary services receiving repeated admissions of service users whose needs are only partially met.

In the next section of this chapter we discuss a politics of recovery, whereby mental health services might be more focused on better serving the needs of users.

A politics of recovery

As we discussed in Chapter 1, within the traditional medical model, healthcare professionals regarded themselves as experts, and therefore saw little value in seeking the views of service users concerning their care. Even in modern mental health services, there remains a degree of disconnection between the staff and service users. This is frustrating as it means that recovery-influenced practice as discussed in earlier chapters is still not having a consistent, positive influence in practice. This sense of 'them and us' is rarely commented upon, but undeniably present in many clinical settings across the country, yet often papered over by the principles of recovery being recited where necessary. This makes the discrepancies between practice and theory all too painfully apparent to students and new practitioners, and is a source of disillusionment to many.

Often recovery is cited as a mantra in mission statements and policies but out in practice bureaucracy, staff shortages, the narrow remits of highly specialist services and agencies not working together all represent barriers to practising in a truly recovery-focused manner. Sceptics suggest that this only goes to prove the limitations of recovery as a flawed concept. A more optimistic way of looking at it might be that our values become even more important and worthwhile where they are tested. If in the face of innumerable challenges we can remain positive, upbeat, hopeful of change and empathic towards our service users, this is the truest indicator that we are practising recovery.

Often students report that they encounter conflicting ideas in practice between the traditional approach and recovery-based models. It is necessary to look more closely at these issues, discuss them openly and to keep the concept of recovery at the centre of our attention.

Exercise

In your practice area, have you ever worked in a service that:

- was slow to respond to people's needs due to staffing shortages/lack of resources; had some staff who lacked motivation, were 'burned out' or cynical?
- had gaps in provision – maybe you wished there were other agencies to which service users could be referred but which did not exist in the locality?
- discharged clients when they seemed 'well enough', but before they were really ready?
- worked with people for only a time-limited period, instead of until their need was met?

1 Write down the examples you have experienced of the above situations.
2 Now write down the factors that you believe contribute to these situations.

None of the above factors mean there is abuse going on, or that a clinical area needs to be shut down. However, the care is not as good as it ought to be. It is often these types of issue that lead to service users feeling dissatisfied. It may be difficult in these circumstances for the service user to articulate their concerns, but nevertheless their needs are not being met as well as they might. This can lead to feelings of alienation or stigmatization within the services tasked with supporting them: the very place that should offer a sense of safety and acceptance.

As we have established, political initiatives have the potential to make a significant impact upon our lives. This is often not appreciated, and perhaps some of our disillusionment with politics is that there is a patent lack of connection between policy and action. As the above exercise suggests, a consistent feature of modern service provision is a lack of resources, lack of co-ordination, and insufficient prioritization of the needs of the individual. That said, it seems to be generally accepted within mental health services that recovery is the way forward, even if the concept is often not well understood. It is undoubtedly the case that aspects of our socio-economic landscape make it difficult for recovery-focused services to become a reality. What is urgently required, and long overdue, is the development of an integrated and unified national mental health strategy, with input from multiple specialists, experts and stakeholders. Within this strategy there needs to be proposals for services from the acute and specialist inpatient sector to the community and mental health promotion. Such a strategy may have the internal coherence and credibility to withstand the buffeting of short-term political initiatives that have often beset the mental health services within the NHS.

What can I do to support the mental health services?

As we discussed in Chapters 4 and 5, self-awareness, reflecting upon practice and examining our motives are essential if we are to make a real difference in practice. Often principles are described in quite broad and vague terms. We know that they refer to positive beliefs and actions and we can say what they are in many cases, such as being fair to everyone and treating all people equally. Yet often such beliefs exist as abstract ideals. Instead they need to be demonstrated and applied in practice where there are competing priorities and genuine ethical dilemmas and no easy answers. Central to embedding a politics of recovery in the mental health nursing workforce is that we really believe it, and implement it, rather than just talk about it. If we return to Chapter 1, we discussed altruism, where care is given in a manner that I would want to receive if I was the service user. The next exercise looks at not only how important it is to do the right thing, but more significantly the motivation and rationale behind our choices.

Exercise

In considering why we care for people who need support with everyday needs, which of the following statements is correct?

Statement A: I think people should be cared for because the state provides support for all of its citizens who require help, and I would hope that help would be there for me.

Statement B: I think people should be cared for because we are all unique feeling individuals and all different. Everyone is important and needs care according to their individual circumstances.

Statement A refers to general principles and standards. It considers my own preferences if I was in that position, and does not look at the person whose needs we are actually meeting, or consider that they are a different and unique individual. However, if the person was initially to resist or refuse help, I might be confused, and perhaps even angry at the person for not accepting help that is appropriate, meets their need and is well-intended. This might be because I am looking at my own feelings and thoughts as opposed to the other person's. In contrast, statement B talks about the needs of the person as a unique individual, and begins from their vantage point as opposed to mine.

It could be argued that both statements have the same outcome, in the sense that the person still receives help and support, only that the reasons are slightly different. Yet these views do produce different results, as if we practised in accordance with statement A, what I might regard as the standard and type of care that I desire might be different than other people. This can lead to 'one-size-fits-all' care, which offers no scope for personal choice or the collaborative development of care. If we practise in accordance with statement B, we will provide care that is flexible and based on the needs of the individual regardless of the circumstances.

Both statements also proceed from quite different political and philosophical backgrounds that are worth considering in greater depth.

Politics begins with us as individuals. As a registered professional your personal accountability and standards for practice are central to your professional role. Having a clear awareness of your principles, and a sense of integrity about articulating these, is important in promoting recovery in practice (NMC, 2015). It is worth investing time and energy to develop your understanding of recovery, and as we discussed in Chapters 1 and 2, working to connect your personal values with the principles of recovery central to mental health nursing practice. You may be required to question and challenge traditional approaches to practise. You will feel more empowered in doing this if you are convinced that recovery is the right approach in practice. This means something to you, as opposed to representing a collection of loose ideas that you know to be right but have not developed a personal commitment towards.

Often institutional practices evolve through habit, lack of thought or just expediency. This can make it difficult to identify a robust rationale for certain practices, or recognize the contribution of some actions to the overall standard of care on the ward. Long-ingrained practices can continue out of a sense of habit and without thought as to the intended purpose of the action. Examples of institutional practices are often negative, but others are harmless or may even seem mildly helpful. For example, as a student nurse on an older people's assessment unit, I was on placement on a number of nights. At the changeover before the night shift, all of the service users were made tea and toast. This was a regimented part of the ward routine. As I was new to the ward, this came as a surprise to me, and the staff were surprised I was surprised. They explained that 'we do that here because we have always done it'. This is a harmless example of an institutional practice, and more noteworthy because of the manner in which the staff rigidly pursued this activity.

However, institutionalized practice can be highly detrimental to the care of service users, as it can obscure opportunities to identify individual needs. In the community, practice can become routine as a result of heavy caseloads. The mental health nurse may be simultaneously assessing the person's mental state, carrying out a risk assessment, and therapeutically engaging with the service user. Reflecting carefully on these multiple roles and the high level of expectation of the practitioner is a useful habit to acquire. This can help you to appreciate the complexity of your role, but also ensures that the service user is listened to and given a response that answers their need. Each interaction is a fresh encounter, which helps to maintain genuine curiosity and interest in service users and their stories (Wrycraft, 2015). This involves looking analytically at the job that we do, and carrying it out creatively, while still doing it thoroughly.

If mental health nurses are to promote positive perceptions of mental health nursing and to combat stigma, it is essential to become involved from a political perspective. Probably the single most influential activity is in your work and personal life, living in a way you would like to be seen, being honest about how you are and how you feel but also to represent the values and beliefs you prioritize. Other actions we can take include:

- joining independent sector organizations that promote mental health;
- working with independent sector organizations, whether in a paid or voluntary capacity;
- volunteering to help at charity events, or taking part in activities to promote positive perceptions and awareness of mental health;
- making posts on websites and online friendship groups to highlight positive perceptions or examples of mental health;
- tactfully challenging instances where people present negative or stereotypical portrayals of people with mental health issues;
- starting up or joining a student mental health nursing society. Often university departments have a small but very useful source of funding available to support student societies;
- starting a journal club with other students or staff on placement areas (see Chapter 5 on clinical supervision);
- other ideas. Can you think of any?

Conclusion

In this chapter we have discussed what politics is, and looked at the current trend of apathy among the electorate. There are reasons for this that are understandable; however, as opposed to continuing to disengage, surely as members of society it demonstrates a recovery approach to become involved with the political process. We looked briefly at the history and development of the NHS, and the role of mental health services within it. Throughout the chapter we have also discussed aspects of Maslow's hierarchy, as these highlight aspects of the extent to which we meet our needs and gain fulfilment.

Provision for mental health is often regarded as lacking parity with physical healthcare services. In spite of government measures to address this issue, there is still scepticism. Without more funding and government commitment to developing a comprehensive policy for mental health, will rhetoric be matched by reality? It is also the case that in recent years following the *NSF for Mental*

Health government policy has been fragmented and provided disparate solutions to different aspects of mental health. The notion of treatment pathways runs counter to individualistic and recovery-oriented care. Such an approach limits the potential for cohesive, responsive, multidisciplinary recovery-based working within mental health services. What is needed is a comprehensive strategy for mental health that, much like the NSF, provides a comprehensive strategy and offers it the same parity as physical health.

Finally in this chapter we looked at a politics of recovery. It is necessary to review, and where necessary challenge, institutional practice. In order for services to fully embody recovery, it is necessary that the attitudes and beliefs of individual practitioners really embrace this concept and implement it within practice.

References

American Psychiatric Association (APA) (2012) *DSM-IV and DSM-5 Criteria for the Personality Disorders*. Available online at: http://www.psi.uba.ar/academica/carrerasdegrado/psicologia/sitios_catedras/practicas_profesionales/820_clinica_tr_personalidad_psicosis/material/dsm.pdf (accessed 12 August 2015).

Andresen, R., Oades, L. and Caputi, P. (2003) The experience of recovery from schizophrenia: towards an empirically validated stage model. *Australian and New Zealand Journal of Psychiatry*, 37, 586–94.

Anthony, W. A. (1993) Recovery from mental illness: the guiding vision of the mental health service system in the 1990s. *Psychosocial Rehabilitation Journal*, 16(4): 11–23.

Anxiety BC (2016) How to do progressive muscle relaxation. Available online at: https://www.anxietybc.com/sites/default/files/MuscleRelaxation.pdf (accessed 7 September, 2016).

Ashmore, R., Carver, N., Clibbens, N. and Sheldon, J. (2012) Lecturers' accounts of facilitating clinical supervision groups within a pre reg mental health nursing curriculum. *Nurse Education Today*, 32(3): 224–8.

Barker, P. (2001) The tidal model: developing an empowering, person-centered approach to recovery within psychiatric and mental health nursing. *Journal of Psychiatric and Mental Health Nursing*, 8(3): 233–40. Available through: Anglia Ruskin University Library website http://libweb.anglia.ac.uk (accessed 3 April 2015).

Barker, P. (2003) The tidal model: psychiatric colonization, recovery and the paradigm shift in mental health care. *International Journal of Mental Health Nursing* [e-journal] 12(2): 96–102. Available through: Anglia Ruskin University Library website http://libweb.anglia.ac.uk (accessed 23 September 2014).

Barker, P. (2008) *Assessment in Psychiatric and Mental Health Nursing*, 2nd edn. Cheltenham: Stanley Thornes Ltd.

Barker, P. J. and Buchanan-Barker, P. (2005) *The Tidal Model: A Guide for Mental Health Professionals*. Hove: Routledge.

Bateman, A. W. and Krawitz, R. (2013) *Borderline Personality Disorder: An Evidence-Based Guide for Generalist Mental Health Professionals*. Oxford: Oxford University Press.

Bond, M. and Holland, S. (2010) *Skills of Clinical Supervision for Nurses*. Maidenhead: McGraw-Hill/Open University Press.

Bonnington, O. and Rose, D. (2014) Exploring stigmatisation among people diagnosed with either bipolar disorder or borderline personality disorder: a critical realist analysis. *Social Science and Medicine* [e-journal], 123(1): 7–17. Available through: Anglia Ruskin University Library website http://libweb.anglia.ac.uk (accessed 8 August 2015).

Borg, M. and Davidson, L. (2008) The nature of recovery as lived in everyday experience. *Journal of Mental Health* [e-journal] 17(2): 129–40. Available through: Anglia Ruskin University Library website http://libweb.anglia.ac.uk (accessed 3 April 2015).

Borrill, C., Carletta, J., Carter, A., Dawson, J., Garrod, S., Rees, A., Richards, A., Shapiro, D. and West, M. (2000) Teamworking and effectiveness in health care: findings from the healthcare team effectiveness project. Available at: http://homepages.inf.ed.ac.uk/jeanc/DOH-glossy-brochure.pdf (accessed 11 September, 2016).

Borton, T. (1970) *Reach, Touch and Teach*. London: Hutchinson.

Boud, D., Keogh, R. and Walker, D. (1985) *Reflection: Turning Experience into Learning*. London: Kogan Page.

British Association for the Person-Centred Approach (2015) *What Is the Person-Centred Approach?* Available at: http://www.bapca.org.uk/ (accessed 6 February 2016).

British Medical Association (BMA) (2014) *Recognising the Importance of Physical Health in Mental Health and Intellectual Disability*. London: BMA.

Buchanan-Barker, P. and Barker, P. J. (2006) The ten commitments: a value base for mental health recovery. *Journal of Psychosocial Nursing and Mental Health Services* [e-journal] 44(9): 29–33. Available through: Anglia Ruskin University Library website http://libweb.anglia.ac.uk (accessed 14 March 2015].

Buchanan-Barker, P. and Barker, P. J. (2008) The tidal commitments: extending the value base of mental health recovery. *Journal of Psychiatric and Mental Health Nursing* [e-journal] 15(2): 93–100. Available through: Anglia Ruskin University Library website http://libweb.anglia.ac.uk (accessed 14 March 2015).

Bulman, C. and Shutz, S. (2013) *Reflective Practice in Nursing*. Chichester: Wiley-Blackwell (ebrary).

Canadian Mental Health Association (2015) *heretohelp: Dealing with a Mental Illness Diagnosis*, p. 3. Toronto: Canadian Mental Health Association. Available online at: http://www.heretohelp.bc.ca/sites/default/files/dealing-with-a-mental-illness-diagnosis.pdf (accessed 22 February 2016).

Carlyle, D., Crowe, M. and Deering, D. (2012) Models of care delivery in mental health nursing practice: a mixed method study. *Journal of Psychiatric and Mental Health Nursing* [e-journal], 19(3): 221–30. Available through Anglia Ruskin University Library website http://libweb.anglia.ac.uk (accessed 23 December 2014).

Catthoor, K., Schrijvers, D., Hutsebaut, J., Feenstra, D. and Sabbe, B. (2015) Psychiatric stigma in treatment-seeking adults with personality problems: evidence from a sample of 214 patients. *Frontiers in Psychiatry* [Abstract]. Available online at: http://www.ncbi.nlm.nih.gov/pubmed/26217243 (accessed 15 March 2016).

Cherry, K. (2017) *What Is Online Therapy? A Look at the Ins and Outs of Online Psychotherapy*. Available online at: http://www.bing.com/search?q=telephone+counselling+in+mental+health&src=IE-TopResult&FORM=IETR02&conversationid= (accessed 13 February 2017).

Chinn, P. L. and Kramer, M. K. (2008) *Integrated Theory and Knowledge Development in Nursing*, 7th edn. St. Louis, MO: Mosby Elsevier.

Clark, D. (2013) 'What is Recovery?' Julie Repper & Rachel Perkins. Available online at: http://www.recoverystories.info/what-is-recovery-julie-repper-rachel-perkins/online (accessed: 29 October 2016).

Coad, A. and Wrycraft, N. (2015) *CBT Approaches for Children and Young People*. Maidenhead: McGraw-Hill/Open University Press.

Coleman, R. (2012) *Recovery: An Alien Concept?* 3rd edn. Port of Ness, Isle of Lewis: P&P Press.

Copeland, M. E. (2014) *WRAP® for Life*. Dummerston: Peach Press.

Copeland, M. E. (2015) *WRAP® Wellness Recovery Action Plan®*. Dummerston: Peach Press.

Crawford, P. and Brown, B. (2009) Mental health communication between service users and professionals: disseminating practice-congruent research. *Mental Health Review*, 14(3): 31–9.

Cutcliffe, J. R., McKenna, H. P., Hyrkäs, K. and Barker, P. J. (2010) *Nursing Models: Application to Practice*. London: Quay.

Davidson, L. (2005) Recovery, self-management and the expert patient – changing the culture of mental health from a UK perspective. *Journal of Mental Health* [e-journal], 14(1): 25–35. Available through: Anglia Ruskin University Library website http://libweb.anglia.ac.uk (accessed 12 January 2015).

Davidson, L., O'Connell, M. J., Tondora, J., Lawless, M. and Evan, A. C. (2005) Recovery in serious mental illness: a new wine or just a new bottle? *Professional Psychology: Research and Practice*, 36: 480–7. Available through: Anglia Ruskin University Library website: http://libweb.anglia.ac.uk (accessed 30 January 2015).

Davidson, L., O'Connell, M., Tondora, J., Styron, T. and Kangas, K. (2006) The top ten concerns about recovery encountered in mental health system transformation. *Psychiatric Services* [e-journal], 57: 640–5. Available through: Anglia Ruskin University Library website http://libweb.anglia.ac.uk (accessed 30 January 2015).

Deegan, P. E. (1988) Recovery: the lived experience of rehabilitation. *Psychosocial Rehabilitation Journal*, 11: 11–19.

Department of Health (DoH) (1999) *The National Service Framework for Mental Health: Modern Standards and Service Models.* Available online at: https://www.gov.uk/government/uploads/system/uploads/attachment_data/file/198051/National_Service_Framework_for_Mental_Health.pdf (accessed: 13 August 2016).

Department of Health (DoH) (2004) *The Ten Essential Shared Capabilities: A Framework for the Whole of the Mental Health Workforce.* [pdf] London: DoH. Available online at: http://www.iapt.nhs.uk/silo/files/10-essential-shared-capabilities.pdf (accessed 8 August 2015).

Department of Health (DoH) (2006) *From Values to Action: The Chief Nursing Officer's Review of Mental Health Nursing.* [pdf]. Available online at: http://webarchive.nationalarchives.gov.uk/20130107105354/http://www.dh.gov.uk/prod_consum_dh/groups/dh_digitalassets/@dh/@en/documents/digitalasset/dh_4133840.pdf (accessed 5 May 2015).

Department of Health (DoH) (2007) *The Essential Shared Capabilities for Practice.* London: DoH.

Department of Health (DoH) (2014) *Achieving Better Access to Mental Health Services by 2020.* Available online at: https://www.gov.uk/government/uploads/system/uploads/attachment_data/file/361648/mental-health-access.pdf (accessed: 16 August 2016).

De-Silva, D. (2011) *Helping People Help Themselves. A Review of the Evidence Considering Whether It Is Worthwhile to Support Self-Management.* London: Health Foundation. Available at: http://www.health.org.uk/sites/default/files/HelpingPeople-HelpThemselves.pdf (accessed 20 January 2016).

Devon Partnership Trust (2014) *Putting Wellbeing at the Heart of Our Recovery.* Exeter: Devon Partnership Trust. Available online at: http://holyford.org/wpcontent/uploads/2014/04/Recovery-Leaflet-daisies-A5-single-pages-final-proof-1.pdf (accessed 29 February 2016).

Drucker, P. (2011) High time for think time. Drucker Institute. Available online at: http://www.druckerinstitute.com/2011/02/high-time-for-think-time/.

Elledge, J. (2014) The Disillusionment Index: Detailing the demise of the big two political parties. Available online at: http://www.may2015.com/parties/the-disillusionment-index-detailing-the-demise-of-the-big-two-political-parties/ (accessed: 27 February 2017).

Engel, G. L. (1977) The need for a new medical model: a challenge for biomedicine. *Science*, 196: 129–36.

Esmiol, E. and Partridge, R. (2014) Enhancing self-awareness using feedback reflection, in R. A. Bean, S. D. Davis and M. P. Davey (eds) *Clinical Supervision Activities for Increasing Competence and Self-Awareness*, Chapter 7, pp. 41–9. Hoboken, NJ: John Wiley and Sons, Inc.

Fallon, P. (2003) Travelling through the system: the lived experience of people with borderline personality disorder in contact with psychiatric services. *Journal of Psychiatric and*

Mental Health Nursing [e-journal], 10(4): 393–400. Available through: Anglia Ruskin University Library website http://libweb.anglia.ac.uk (accessed 2 August 2015).

Falvey, M., Forest, M., Pearpoint, J. and Rosenberg, R. (2000) *All My Life's a Circle: Using the Tools: Circles, MAPS and PATH*. Toronto: Inclusion Press.

Fawcett, J. (1995) *Analysis and Evaluation of Conceptual Models of Nursing*, 3rd edn. Philadelphia, PA: F. A. Davis.

Fawcett, J. (2005) *Contemporary Nursing Knowledge: Analysis and Evaluation of Nursing Models and Theories*, 2nd edn. Philadelphia: F. A. Davis.

Filer, N. (2005) Borderline personality disorder: attitudes of mental health nurses. *Mental Health Practice* [e-journal], 9(2): 34–6. Available through: Anglia Ruskin University Library website http://libweb.anglia.ac.uk (accessed 8 August 2015).

Forchuk, D. (1993) *Hildegard E. Peplau: Interpersonal Nursing Theory*. London: Sage Publications.

Foucault, M. (1989) *Madness and Civilization: A History of Insanity in the Age of Reason*. London: Routledge.

Freire, P. (2005) *Pedagogy of the Oppressed*. New York: The Continuum International Publishing Group Inc.

Freshwater, D. (2002) *Therapeutic Nursing: Improving Patient Care through Self-Awareness and Reflection*. London: Sage Publications.

Gillespie, M. (2010) Relapse in long term conditions: learning from mental health methods. *British Journal of Nursing*, 19(19): 1236–42.

Goffman, E. (1961) *Asylums: On the Social Situation of Mental Patients and Other Inmates*. New York: First Anchor Press.

Gournay, K. (1995) What to do with nursing models. *Journal of Psychiatric and Mental Health Nursing* [e-journal], 2(5): 325–7. Available through: Anglia Ruskin University Library website: http://libweb.anglia.ac.uk (accessed 14 February 2015).

Gournay, K. (1997) Responses to: 'What to do with nursing models' – a reply from Gournay. *Journal of Psychiatric and Mental Health Nursing* [e-journal], 4(3): 227–31. Available through: Anglia Ruskin University Library website: http://libweb.anglia. ac.uk (accessed 4 March 2015).

GOV.UK (2014) Making mental health as important as physical health. Available online at: https://www.gov.uk/government/news/making-mental-health-as-important-as-physical-health (accessed: 27 February 2017).

Grosjean, B. and G. E. Tsai (2007) NMDA neurotransmission as a critical mediator of borderline personality disorder. *Journal of Psychiatry and Neuroscience* [e-journal] 32(2): 103–13. Available through: Anglia Ruskin University Library website http://libweb.anglia.ac.uk (accessed 13 August 2015).

Hartweg, D. L. (1991) *Dorothea Orem: Self-Care Deficit Theory of Nursing*. London: Sage Publications.

Hawkins, P. and Shohet, R. (2012) *Supervision in the Helping Professions*. Maidenhead: McGraw-Hill/Open University Press.

Healy, D. and McSharry, P. (2011) Promoting self-awareness in undergraduate nursing students in relation to their health status and personal behaviours. *Nurse Education in Practice*, 11(4): 228–33.

Heidegger, M. (2003) *Being and Time*. Oxford: Blackwell Publishing Ltd.

Heron, J. (2001) *Helping the Client*. London: Sage Publications.

Hierarchy of Needs (2014) [Image] Available online at: http://psed516diversityproject. wikispaces.com/file/view/Hierarchyofneeds.jpg/385872838/Hierarchyofneeds.jpg (accessed 10 May 2014).

HM Government (1998) *The Data Protection Act*. Available online at: http://www.legislation. gov.uk/ukpga/1998/29/pdfs/ukpga_19980029_en.pdf (accessed 30 March 2017).

HM Government (2003) *The Victoria Climbie Inquiry.* Available online at: https://www.gov.uk/government/uploads/system/uploads/attachment_data/file/273183/5730.pdf (accessed: 27 March 2017).

HM Government (2007) *The Mental Health Act.* Available online at: http://www.legislation.gov.uk/ukpga/2007/12/pdfs/ukpga_20070012_en.pdf (accessed 17 July 2016).

HM Government (2011) *No Health Without Mental Health: A Cross-Government Mental Health Outcomes Strategy for People of All Ages.* Available online at: https://www.gov.uk/government/uploads/system/uploads/attachment_data/file/213761/dh_124058.pdf (accessed 16 August 2016).

Horn, N., Johnstone, L. and Brooke, S. (2007) Some service user perspectives on the diagnosis of Borderline Personality Disorder. *Journal of Mental Health* [e-journal], 16(20): 255–69. Available through: Anglia Ruskin University Library website http://libweb.anglia.ac.uk (accessed 2 August 2015).

http://www.express.co.uk/news/politics/645667/Brexit-EU-European-Union-Referendum-David-Cameron-Economic-Impact-UK-EU-exit-leave (accessed 27 February 2017).

http://www.mhpf.org.uk/sites/default/files/documents/publications/mhpfuserguide_v2.pdf (accessed: 7 September 2016).

Jankovic, J., Richards, F. and Priebe, S. (2010) Advance statements in adult mental health. *Advances in Psychiatric Treatment*, 16: 448–55. Available online at: doi: to 10.1192/apt.bp.109.006932.

Jeffers, S. (2011) *Feel the Fear and Do It Anyway.* London: Arrow Books.

Jenkins, R. and Elliott, P. (2004) Stressors, burnout and social support: nurses in acute mental health settings. *Journal of Advanced Nursing*, 48(6): 622–31.

Johns, C. (2013) *Becoming A Reflective Practitioner.* Chichester: Wiley-Blackwell.

Jones, A. (1996) The value of Peplau's theory for mental health nursing. *British Journal of Nursing* [e-journal], 5(14): 877–81. Available through: Anglia Ruskin University Library website http://libweb.anglia.ac.uk (accessed 14 March 2015).

Jones, K. (1993) *Asylums and After: A Revised History of the Mental Health Services from the Early 18th Century to the 1990s.* London: The Athlone Press.

Jowitt, J. (2012) British democracy in terminal decline, warns report. Available online at: https://www.theguardian.com/uk/2012/jul/06/british-democracy-decline-report (accessed: 27 February 2017).

Kabat-Zin, J. (1990/2013) *Full Catastrophe Living: How to Cope with Stress, Pain and Illness Using Mindfulness Meditation.* London: Piatkus.

Ke, M. K., Blazeby, J. M., Strong, S., Carroll, F. E., Ness, A. R. and Hollingworth, W. (2013) Are multidisciplinary teams in secondary care cost-effective? A systematic review of the literature. *Cost Effectiveness and Resource Allocation*, 11: 7. Available online at: http://resource-allocation.biomedcentral.com/articles/10.1186/1478-7547-11-7 (accessed: 29 March 2017).

King's Fund (2013) *The Francis Report.* Available online at: www.kingsfund.org.uk/Francis-Report.

King's Fund (2016) 'Has the government put mental health on an equal footing with physical health?' Available online at: http://www.kingsfund.org.uk/projects/verdict/has-government-put-mental-health-equal-footing-physical-health (accessed 16 August 2016).

Kiume, S. (2013). Top 10 Mental Health Apps. Psych Central. Available online at: https://psychcentral.com/blog/archives/2013/01/16/top-10-mental-health-apps/ (accessed 13 February 2017).

Kolb, D. A. (1984) *Experiential Learning: Experience as a Source of Learning and Development.* Englewood Cliffs, NJ: Prentice Hall.

Laing, R. D. (1970) *The Divided Self.* London: Penguin.

Legislation.gov.uk. (1983) *Mental Health Act 1983.* [pdf] London: Legislation. gov.uk. Available online at: http://www.legislation.gov.uk/ukpga/1983/20/pdfs/ukpga_ 19830020_en.pdf (accessed 10 August 2015).

Legislation.gov.uk. (2007) *Mental Health Act 2007.* [pdf] London: Legislation.gov.uk. Available online at: http://www.legislation.gov.uk/ukpga/2007/12/pdfs/ukpga_20070012_ en.pdf (accessed 9 August 2015).

Link, B. G., Cullen, F. T., Frank, J. and Wozniak, J. F. (1987) The social rejection of former mental patients: understanding why labels matter. *American Journal of Sociology* [e-journal] 92(6): 1461–500. Available through: Anglia Ruskin University Library website http://libweb.anglia.ac.uk (accessed 7 August 2015).

Local Safeguarding Children Board (LSCB) Haringey (2009) Available online at: http:// www.haringeylscb.org/sites/haringeylscb/files/executive_summary_peter_final.pdf (accessed: 27 March 2017).

Longden, E. (2011) *Knowing You, Knowing You* [DVD]. Port of Ness, Isle of Lewis: Working to Recovery Ltd.

MacKeith, J. and Burns, S. (2011) *User Guide: Mental Health Recovery Star.* Available online at: www.amazon.co.uk/Mental-Health-Recovery-Star-Guide/dp10955919606.

Markham, D. (2003) Attitudes towards patients with a diagnosis of borderline personality disorder: social rejection and dangerousness. *Journal of Mental Health* [e-journal], 12(6): 595–612. Available through: Anglia Ruskin University Library website http:// libweb.anglia.ac.uk (accessed 7 August 2015).

Marmot Review (2010) *Fair Society, Healthy Lives: The Marmot Review Executive Summary.* Available at: http://www.bing.com/search?q=Fair+Society+Healthy+Live s+PDF&FORM=R5FD6 (accessed 16 August 2016).

Maslow, A. H. (1943) A theory of human motivation. *Psychological Review*, 50(4): 370–96.

Maslow, A. H. (1954) *Motivation and Personality.* New York: Harper & Row.

McAllister, M. and Moyle, W. (2008) An exploration of mental health nursing models of care in a Queensland psychiatric hospital. *International Journal of Mental Health Nursing* [e-journal], 17(1): 18–26. Available through: Anglia Ruskin University Library website http://libweb.anglia.ac.uk (accessed 13 February 2015).

McKenna, H. (1997) *Nursing Theories and Models.* London: Routledge.

McKenna, H. P. (2014) *Fundamentals of Nursing Models, Theories and Practice,* 2nd edn. Chichester: Wiley-Blackwell.

McKenna, H. P. and Slevin, O. (2008) *Nursing Models, Theories and Practice.* Chichester: Blackwell Publishing.

McLeod, S. A. (2014) *Maslow's Hierarchy of Needs.* Available online at: www.simplypsy- chology.org/maslow.html (accessed 28 March 2016).

Medical Research Council (MRC) (2016) Study finds virtual reality can help treat severe paranoia. Available at: https://www.mrc.ac.uk/news/browse/study-finds-virtual-reality- can-help-treat-severe-paranoia/ (accessed 13 February, 2017).

Mental Health Foundation (MHF) (2007) *The Fundamental Facts: The Latest Facts and Figures on Mental Health.* London: MHF.

Mental Health Foundation (MHF) (2011) *Physical Health and Mental Health.* Available online at: www.mentalhealth.org.uk/our-work/policy/physical-health-and-mental-health (accessed 14 November 2014).

Mental Health Foundation (MHF) (2015) *Physical Health and Mental Health.* Available online at: http://www.mentalhealth.org.uk/help-information/mental-health-a-z/P/ physical-health-mental-health/ (accessed 17 November 2015).

Mental Health Taskforce (2016) *The Five Year Forward View for Mental Health: A Report from the Independent Mental Health Taskforce to the NHS in England.* Available online at: https://www.england.nhs.uk/wp-content/uploads/2016/02/Mental-Health-Taskforce-FYFV-final.pdf (accessed: 19 September 2016).

Mind (2011) *Listening to Experience: An Independent Inquiry into Acute and Crisis Mental Healthcare*. London: Mind. Available online at: http://www.mind.org.uk/media/211306/listening_to_experience_web.pdf (accessed 7 August 2015).

Mind (2012) *Personality Disorders*. Available online at: http://www.mind.org.uk/information-support/types-of-mental-health-problems/personality-disorders/.VGDm1fmsUdo (accessed 8 August 2015).

Mind (2015) *Understanding Borderline Personality Disorder*. London: Mind. Available online at: http://www.mind.org.uk/media/2198702/understanding-bpd-2015-online-version.pdf (accessed 13 August 2015).

National Institute for Health and Care Excellence (NICE) (2009) *Borderline Personality Disorder: Treatment and Management*. Available online at: /www.nice.org.uk/guidance/cg78/chapter/key-priorities-for-implementation (accessed 13 August 2015).

National Standards for Mental Health Practice (2010) *Principles of Recovery Orientated Practice*. Available online at: www.health.gov.au/internet/main/publishing.nsf/Content/CFA833CB8C1AA178CA257BF0001E7520/$File/servpri.pdf.

Neuman, B. (1995) *The Neuman Systems Model*. Norwalk, CT: Appleton & Lange.

NHS (2012) *The NHS Constitution*. Available online at: www.gov.uk/government/publications/the-nhs-constitution-for-england.

NHS (2015) *The NHS Constitution: The NHS Belongs to All*. Available online at: https://www.gov.uk/government/uploads/system/uploads/attachment_data/file/480482/NHS_Constitution_WEB.pdf (accessed 17 July 2016).

NHS Choices (2015) *The Care Programme Approach*. Available online at: http://www.nhs.uk/Conditions/social-care-and-support-guide/Pages/care-programme-approach.aspx (accessed 19 September 2016).

NHS Education for Scotland (2011) *The 10 Essential Shared Capabilities for Mental Health Practice: Learning Materials (Scotland)*. Edinburgh: www.nes.scot.nhs.uk.

NHS England (2013) *Transforming Participation in Health and Care: The NHS Belongs to Us All*. England: NHS England. Available at: www.england.nhs.uk/wp-content/uploads/2013/09/trans-part-hc-guid1.pdf (accessed 7 August 2015).

NHS England (2014) *MDT Development – Working Toward an Effective Multidisciplinary/Multiagency Team* [pdf]. Available online at: www.england.nhs.uk/wp-content/uploads/2015/01/mdt-dev-guid-flat-fin.pdf (accessed 2 October 2015).

NHS England (2015) *MDT Development – Working Toward an Effective Multidisciplinary/Multiagency Team*. Available online at: https://www.england.nhs.uk/wp-content/uploads/2015/01/mdt-dev-guid-flat-fin.pdf (accessed 11 September 2016).

NHS England (2016) *Implementing the Five Year Forward View for Mental Health*. London: England.

NHS England (2017) *Implementing the Five Year Forward View for Mental Health*. London: NHS England. Gateway Reference: 05575.

Nolan, P. (1993) *A History of Mental Health Nursing*. London: Chapman and Hall.

Norfolk, Suffolk and Cambridgeshire Strategic Heallth Authority (2003) Independent inquiry into the death of David Bennett. Available online at: http://image.guardian.co.uk/sys-files/Society/documents/2004/02/12/Bennett.pdf (accessed 23 February 2017).

Norman, I. and Ryrie, I. (2013) *The Art and Science of Mental Health Nursing: Principles and Practice*, 3rd edn. Maidenhead: McGraw-Hill/Open University Press.

Nurseslabs (2016) *Dorothea Orem's Self Care Theory*. Available online at: https://nurseslabs.com/dorothea-orems-self-care-theory/.

Nursing and Midwifery Council (NMC) (2015) *The Code: Professional Standards of Practice and Behaviour for Nurses and Midwives*. London: NMC. Available online at: http://www.nmc-uk.org/Documents/NMC-Publications/NMC-Code-A5-FINAL.pdf (accessed 7 August 2015).

Nursing and Midwifery Council (NMC) (2016) Welcome to revalidation. Available online at: http://revalidation.nmc.org.uk/welcome-to-revalidation (accessed 9 August 2016).

Nursing Theory (2016) Self-care deficit theory. Available online at: http://nursing-theory.org/theories-and-models/orem-self-care-deficit-theory.php (accessed 24 February 2017).

O'Brien, J., Pearpoint, J. and Kahn, L. (2012) *The PATH and MAPS Handbook. Person-Centred Ways to Build Community.* Toronto: Inclusion Press.

Paris, J. and Zweig-Frank, H. (2001) A 27-year follow-up of patients with borderline personality disorder. *Comprehensive Psychiatry* [e-journal], 42(6): 482–7. Available through: Anglia Ruskin University Library website http://libweb.anglia.ac.uk (accessed 13 August 2015).

Pearpoint, J. (2015) *Background – PATH.* Available online at: jack@inclusion.com.Wed 09/09/2015 15:19 (accessed 23 September 2015).

Pearson, A., Vaughan, B. and FitzGerald, M. (2005) *Nursing Models for Practice*, 3rd edn. New York: Butterworth-Heinemann.

Peplau, H. (1952) *Interpersonal Relations in Nursing.* New York: Putnam.

Peplau, H. E. (1988) *Interpersonal Relations in Nursing: A Conceptual Framework of Reference for Psychodynamic Nursing.* New York: Springer.

Perkins, R. and Repper, J. (2013) Prejudice, discrimination and social exclusion: reducing the barriers to recovery for people diagnosed with mental health problems in the UK. *Neuropsychiatry* [e-journal], 3(4): 377–84. Available through: Anglia Ruskin University Library website http://libweb.anglia.ac.uk (accessed 22 May 2015).

Pierret, C. R. (2006) The 'sandwich generation': women caring for parents and children. Available online at: http://www.bls.gov/opub/mlr/2006/09/art1full.pdf (accessed 16 September 2016).

Proctor, B. (2008) *Group Supervision: A Guide to Creative Practice.* London: Sage Publications.

Pryjmachuk, S. (2011) Theoretical perspectives in mental health nursing: a source of information, in S. Pryjmachuk (ed.) *Mental Health Nursing: An Evidence-Based Introduction*, Chapters 1–3. London: Sage Publications.

Repper, J. and Perkins, R. (2003) *Social Inclusion and Recovery: A Model for Mental Health Practice.* Edinburgh: Baillière Tindall.

Rethink (2013) *Would You Tell? Opening Up about Schizoprenia* [pdf]. London: Rethink. Available online at: https://www.rethink.org/media/858268/Rethink%20Mental%20Illness%20-%20would%20you%20tell%20report.pdf (accessed 17 November 2015).

Rethink: AstraZeneca (2010) *Recovery Insights: Learning from Lived Experience. Rethink Recovery*, vol. 3. London: Rethink.

Rethink Mental Illness (2010) *Recovery Insights: Learning from Lived Experience.* London: Rethink Mental Illness.

Roberts, G. and Boardman, J. (2014) Becoming a recovery oriented practitioner. *Advances in Psychiatric Treatment*, 20: 37–47.

Rodgers, M., Asaria, M., Walker, S., McMillan, D., Lucock, M., Harden, M., Palmer, S. and Eastwood, A. (2012) The clinical effectiveness and cost-effectiveness of low-intensity psychological interventions for the secondary prevention of relapse after depression: a systematic review. *Health Technology Assessment*, 16(28), ISSN 1366-5278.

Rolfe, G. (2001) Models of critical reflection, in G. Rolfe, M. Jasper and D. Freshwater (eds) *Critical Reflection in Practice: Generating Knowledge for Care*, 2nd edn. Basingstoke: Palgrave Macmillan.

Romme, M. and Escher, S. (2000) *Making Sense of Voices: The Mental Health Professional's Guide to Working with Voice-Hearers.* London: Mind.

Romme, M., Escher, S., Dillon, J., Corstens, D. and Morris, M. (2011) *Living with Voices: Fifty Stories of Recovery.* Ross-on-Wye: PCCS Books.

Roper, N., Logan, W. and Tierney, A. J. (2000) *The Roper-Logan-Tierney Model of Nursing: Based on Activities of Living.* Edinburgh: Churchill-Livingstone.

Royal College of Psychiatrists (RCP) (2010) No health without public mental health: the case for action, RCP position statement PS4/2010. Available online at: http://www.rcpsych.ac.uk/PDF/Position%20Statement%204%20website.pdf (accessed 9 April 2015).

Rycroft-Malone, J. and Bucknall, T. (2010) *Models and Frameworks for Implementing Evidence-Based Practice: Linking Evidence to Action.* Chichester: Wiley-Blackwell.

Schmahl, C., Herpertz, S. C., Bertsch, K., Ended, G., Flor, H. and Kirsch, P. (2014) *Mechanisms of Disturbed Emotion Processing and Social Interaction in Borderline Personality Disorder: State of Knowledge and Research Agenda of the German Clinical Research Unit* [online]. Available at: www.ncbi.nim.nih.gov/NCBI/Literature/PubMed. Central (PMC).

Schön, D. (2008) *The Reflective Practitioner: How Professionals Think in Action.* New York: Basic Books.

Sen, P. and Irons, A. (2010) *Personality Disorder and the Mental Health Act 1983 (Amended).* Available online at: http://apt.rcpsych.org/content/16/5/329.full (accessed 9 January 2015).

Senivassen, A. (2016) Journal Club (SEPT intranet).

Sheenan, L., Nieweglowski. K. and Corrigan. P. (2016) The stigma of personality disorders. *Current Psychiatry Reports*, 18(1) [Abstract]. Available online at: http://www.ncbi.nlm.nih.gov/pubmed/26780206 (accessed 15 March 2016).

Shepherd, G., Boardman, J. and Slade, M. (2008) *Making Recovery a Reality* [e-book]. London: The Sainsbury Centre for Mental Health. Available through: Anglia Ruskin University Library website http://libweb.anglia.ac.uk (accessed 12 November 2014).

Skinner, V. and Wrycraft, N. (2014) *CBT Fundamentals: Theory and Cases.* Maidenhead: McGraw-Hill/Open University Press.

Slade, M. (2009) *100 Ways to Support Recovery: A Guide for Mental Health Professionals.* London: Rethink. www.rethink.org/research.

Slade, M. (2013) *100 Ways to Support Recovery: A Guide for Professionals.* London: Rethink Mental Illness.

Stacey, G. and Stickley, T. (2012) Recovery as a threshold concept in mental health nurse education. *Nurse Education Today*, 32: 534–9.

Stevenson, C. and Fletcher, E. (2002) The tidal model: the questions answered. *Mental Health Practice* [e-journal], 5(8): 29–37. Available through: Google scholar, Anglia Ruskin University Library website http://libweb.anglia.ac.uk (accessed 14 March 2015).

Szasz T. S. (2000) Curing the therapeutic state: Thomas Szasz on the medicalisation of American life. Interviewed by Jacob Sullum. *Reason*, 20 July, pp. 27–34. Available through: Anglia Ruskin University Library website http://libweb.anglia.ac.uk (accessed 20 June 2015).

Szasz, T. S. (2010) *The Myth of Mental Illness: Foundations of a Theory of Personal Conduct.* London: Harper & Row.

The Centre of Excellence in Interdisciplinary Mental Health (CEIMH), University of Birmingham and Birmingham & Solihull Mental Health (BSMHT) NHS Trust (2008) *A Recovery Approach to Mental Health Care, Using the Tidal Model: Turning the Tide Handbook.* Available online at: http://www.birmingham.ac.uk/Documents/college-social-sciences/social-policy/CEIMH/Tidal-model-handbook.pdf (accessed 14 March 2015).

The Schizophrenia Commission (2012) *The Abandoned Illness: A Report from the Schizophrenia Commission*. London: Rethink Mental Illness.

Thomas, N., Stainton, T., Jackson, S., Wai Yee, C., Doubtfire, S. and Webb, A. (2003) 'Your friends don't understand': invisibility and unmet need in the lives of 'young carers'. *Child and Family Social Work*, 8: 35–46. Available online at: http://web.a.ebscohost.com/ehost/pdfviewer/pdfviewer?sid=592d6a00-7ec3-4e56-87f3-2ad9ab30c729%40sessionmgr4009&vid=1&hid=4212 (accessed 16 September 2016).

Thomson, G. D. L. (2010) *Personality Disorder and Mental Health Legislation in the UK: Commentary on . . . Personality Disorder and the Mental Health Act 1983 (Amended)*. Available online at: http://apt.rcpsych.org/content/16/5/336.full (accessed 9 August 2015).

Triggle, N. (2014) *Chief Medical Officer: Make Mental Health a Bigger Priority*. Available online at: http://www.bbc.co.uk/news/health-29116354 (accessed 13 August 2016).

Tucker, I. (2010) Mental health service user territories: enacting 'safe spaces' in the community. *Health* [e-journal], 14(4): 434–48. Available through: Anglia Ruskin University Library website http://libweb.anglia.ac.uk (accessed 23 December 2014).

Tyrer, P. (2009) Why borderline personality disorder is neither borderline nor a personality disorder. *Personality and Mental Health*, 3(2): 86–95.

UK Government (2012) *Health and Social Care Act*. Available online at: http://www.legislation.gov.uk/ukpga/2012/7/pdfs/ukpga_20120007_en.pdf (accessed 16 August 2016).

UK Political Info (2016) General election turnout 1945–2015. Available online at: http://www.ukpolitical.info/Turnout45.htm (accessed 13 November 2016).

Wahl, O. and Aroesty-Cohen, E. (2010) Attitudes of mental health professionals about mental illness: a review of the recent literature. *Journal of Community Psychology* [e-journal] 38(1): 48–62. Available through: Anglia Ruskin University Library website http://libweb.anglia.ac.uk (accessed 7 January 2015).

Weinstein, J. (2010) *Mental Health, Service User Involvement and Recovery*. London: Jessica Kingsley Publishers.

Williams, A. (2014) Therapeutic communication in mental health nursing, in S. Walker (ed.) *Engagement and Therapeutic Communication in Mental Health Nursing*, Chapter 1, pp. 5–23. London: Sage: Learning Matters.

Williams, M. and Penman, D. (2011) *Mindfulness: A Practical Guide to Finding Peace in a Frantic World*. London: Piatkus.

Wix, S. and Humphrys, M. (2005) *Working in Forensic Mental Health Care*. London: Elsevier: Churchill Livingstone.

World Health Organization (WHO) (2010) *The ICD-10 Classification of Mental and Behavioural Disorders*. [pdf] Geneva, CH: WHO. Available at: http://www.who.int/classifications/icd/en/bluebook.pdf (accessed 13 August 2015).

Wright, N. and Stickley, T. (2013) Concepts of social inclusion, exclusion and mental health: a review of the international literature. *Journal of Psychiatric and Mental Health Nursing* [e-journal], 20(1): 71–81. Available through: Anglia Ruskin University Library website http://libweb.anglia.ac.uk (accessed 23 December 2014).

Wrycraft, N. (ed.) (2009) *Introduction to Mental Health Nursing*, Chapter 2. Maidenhead: McGraw-Hill/Open University Press.

Wrycraft, N. (2012) *Mental Health Nursing: Case Book*. Maidenhead: McGraw-Hill/Open University Press.

Wrycraft, N. (2015) *Assessment and Care Planning in Mental Health Nursing*. Maidenhead: McGraw-Hill Education/Open University Press.

Zubin, J. and Spring, B. (1977) Vulnerability – a new view of schizophrenia. *Journal of Abnormal Psychology*, 86(2): 103–24.

Index

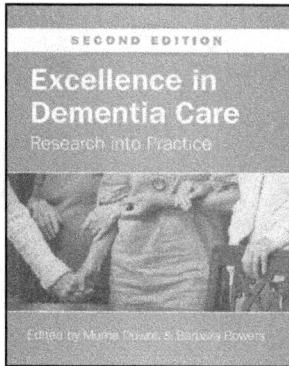

Excellence in Dementia Care
Principles and Practices
Second Edition

Downs and Bowers

ISBN: 9780335245338 (Paperback)
eBook: 9780335245345
2014

This scholarly yet accessible textbook is the most comprehensive single text in the field of dementia care. Drawn from research evidence, international expertise and good practice guidelines, the book has been crafted alongside people with dementia and their families. Case studies and quotes in every chapter illustrate the realities of living with dementia and bring the theory to life.

Key topics include:

- Dementia friendly communities
- Representations of dementia in the media
- Younger people with dementia
- The arts and dementia
- Whole person assessment
- Dementia friendly physical design
- Transitions in care
- Enhancing relationships between families and those with dementia

www.openup.co.uk

OPEN UNIVERSITY PRESS
McGraw · Hill Education

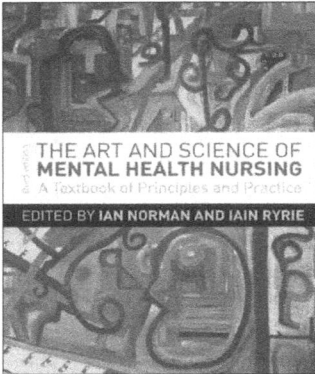

THE ART AND SCIENCE OF MENTAL HEALTH NURSING
A Textbook of Principles and Practice
Third Edition

Ian Norman and Iain Ryrie

ISBN: 9780335245611 (Paperback)
eBook: 9780335245628
2013

This well-established textbook is a must buy for all mental health nursing students. Comprehensive and broad, it explores in detail the many ways in which mental health nursing can have a positive impact on the lives of those with mental health problems. This book includes pedagogy to help students get the most out of each chapter and apply theory to practice in a rewarding way

Key features:

- **Case Studies:** Based on real practice in a variety of settings
- **Thinking Space:** These will help you reflect on your practice and assess your learning
- **Quotes from service users:** These offer the service user perspective throughout the book

www.openup.co.uk

OPEN UNIVERSITY PRESS
McGraw - Hill Education

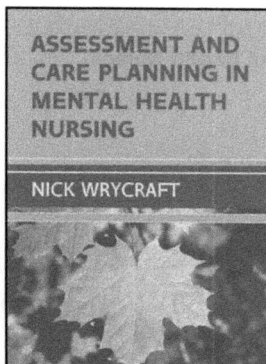

ASSESSMENT AND
CARE PLANNING IN
MENTAL HEALTH
NURSING

NICK WRYCRAFT

Assessment and Care Planning in Mental Health
Nursing

Nick Wrycraft

ISBN: 9780335262984 (Paperback)
eBook: 9780335262991
2015

Assessment of mental health problems is a challenging area of practice that covers a range of symptoms and behaviours – and involves building a trusting relationship with the service user while also using specialist skills. Care planning involves translating information emerging from assessment to collaboratively identify goals and aspirations that are meaningful yet also realistic and personalized.

The first section of the book explores core aspects of assessment including communication skills and engaging the service user before considering risk assessment, care planning, interventions, relapse prevention and reflection. The next section will be ideal for quick reference during practice and looks at 23 different clinical behaviours that nurses will assess, under 4 categories:

Physical factors in mental health
Behavioural aspects in mental health
The role of thoughts in mental health
Feelings in mental health

www.mheducation.co.uk

OPEN UNIVERSITY PRESS
McGraw - Hill Education

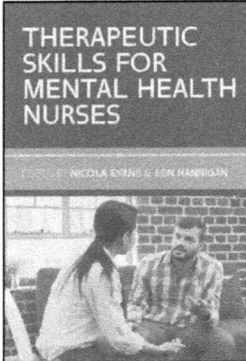

THERAPEUTIC
SKILLS FOR
MENTAL HEALTH
NURSES

NICOLA EVANS & BEN HANNIGAN

Therapeutic Skills for Mental Health Nurses

Evans and Hannigan

ISBN: 9780335264407 (Paperback)
eISBN: 9780335264414

2016

Most specialist mental health care is provided by nurses who use face-to-face
helping skills with a wide range of people in a variety of contexts. This book
puts therapeutic skills at the heart of the nurse's role, with one central aim: to
equip you with knowledge to use in your practice, thus improving your ability to
deliver care.

This book:

- Will enable you to strengthen your core therapeutic skills and broaden
  your knowledge to include other practical therapeutic approaches
- Collates in one place information on a range of therapeutic approaches,
  from person centred counselling, motivational interviewing and solution
  focused approaches, through to day-to-day skills of challenging unhelpful
  thoughts, de-escalating difficult situations, working with families, and
  problem solving
- Demonstrates application of theory to practice through a variety of
  practical examples
- Features reader activities to facilitate personal growth and learning
- Includes a chapter exploring clinical supervision and how this makes
  practice more effective

www.mheducation.co.uk

OPEN UNIVERSITY PRESS
McGraw - Hill Education